Eating and Drinking
in Labour

Commissioning editor: Mary Seager
Desk editor: Deena Burgess
Production controller: Chris Jarvis
Development editor: Caroline Savage
Cover designer: Fred Rose

Eating and Drinking in Labour

Edited by

Penny Champion MSc Advanced Midwifery Practice, ADM, RM, RN
and
Carol McCormick PGDip Law, BSc (Hons), ADM, RM, RN

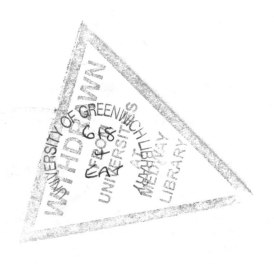

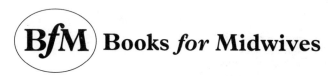

BfM **Books *for* Midwives**

OXFORD AUCKLAND BOSTON JOHANNESBURG MELBOURNE NEW DELHI

Books for Midwives
An imprint of Butterworth-Heinemann
Linacre House, Jordan Hill, Oxford OX2 8DP
225 Wildwood Avenue, Woburn, MA 01801-2041
A division of Reed Educational and Professional Publishing Ltd

℞ A member of the Reed Elsevier plc group

First published 2002

British Library Cataloguing in Publication Data
Champion, Penny
    Eating and drinking in labour
    1. Labour (Obstetrics)   2. Ingestion
    I. Title   II. McCormick, Carol
    618.4

ISBN 0 7506 5315 9 √srb

For information on all Butterworth-Heinemann publications visit
our website at www.bh.com

Typeset by Avocet Typeset, Brill, Aylesbury, Bucks
Printed and bound in Great Britain by Biddles Ltd, Guildford and Kings Lynn

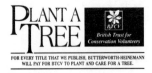

PLANT A
TREE

*British Trust for
Conservation Volunteers*

FOR EVERY TITLE THAT WE PUBLISH, BUTTERWORTH-HEINEMANN
WILL PAY FOR BTCV TO PLANT AND CARE FOR A TREE.

Contents

Contributors   vii

Preface   ix

1   The childbearing continuum: what are the issues around food and drink for labouring women?   1
Penny Champion and Carol McCormick

2   Cultural and historical perspectives on eating and drinking in labour   10
Carol McCormick and Penny Champion

3   Labouring over food: the dietician's view   29
Ann Micklewright and Penny Champion

4   Changes in maternal food appetite and metabolism in labour and the shift from fetal to neonatal metabolism   46
Mary McNabb

5   Eating and drinking in labour: the consumer's view   111
Louise Pengelley

6   Putting the evidence into practice   124
Penny Champion and Carol McCormick

Appendix
Nottingham City Hospital Policy Guidelines for Feeding Women in Labour   137

Index   145

Life is the art of drawing sufficient conclusions from
insufficient premises

Samuel Butler

Contributors

Penny Champion MSc Advanced Midwifery Practice, ADM, RM, RN
Midwifery Lecturer, Anglia Polytechnic University, Midwifery and Human Sexuality Division

Carol McCormick PGDip Law, BSc (Hons), ADM, RM, RN
Midwife, Nottingham City Hospital

Mary McNabb RM, RN, ADM, PGCEA, BSc, BA, MSc
Senior Lecturer, Postgraduate Midwifery Education, South Bank University

Ann Micklewright MSc, SRD
Dietetic and Nutrition Service Manager, Queens Medical Centre, Nottingham; Special Lecturer, School of Biomedical Science, University of Nottingham

Louise Pengelley BA
National Childbirth Trust antenatal teacher and tutor

Preface

The issue of whether women should have the choice of eating and drinking in labour is a contentious one. Many specialists, including midwives, obstetricians, anaesthetists, physiologists, specialist nurses and consumer group experts, have written about their views or the results of research relevant to this issue. However there is no consensus of opinion. This situation makes it very difficult for practising midwives and other practitioners in maternity care to help women make an informed decision about eating and drinking in labour.

The current climate, which upholds women's choice, lends itself to a book offering a review of the research and literature available regarding eating and drinking in labour. As practising midwives ourselves, we feel it would be a valuable guide to our colleagues in helping them to facilitate a more balanced and informed choice with childbearing women.

Relevant information regarding this subject is found in a diverse and sometimes inaccessible selection of books and journals. It is not always possible for an individual practitioner to gather all the relevant literature in order to be fully informed about practice. Therefore the aim of this book is to draw together recent and useful information with a view to assessing the gaps in our knowledge which need to be filled in order to develop pertinent midwifery practice and midwifery research in the future.

CHAPTER ONE

The childbearing continuum: what are the issues around food and drink for labouring women?

Penny Champion and Carol McCormick

- Poor historical evidence to support current practice
- The importance of implementing the recommendations from the Confidential Enquiries into Maternal Mortality
- Multidisciplinary adherence to anaesthetic guidelines of paramount importance
- Medicalization of childbirth – effects on women and midwives
- The need to re-examine practice

The childbearing continuum

The subject we are exploring in this book tends to concentrate the mind on the woman in labour. As practitioners in maternity care, we have responsibility for the care of the childbearing woman, from the time she chooses to seek our care to 28 days after the birth of her child. It is important therefore to look not only at the detailed picture of labour and delivery, but also at the broader spectrum of the childbearing continuum. The physiological approach explored in Chapter 4 of this book highlights this issue. We cannot single out the time of labour from the whole physiological preparation for childbearing, and equally we cannot forget the psychological issues which surround the very significant social events of eating and drinking. It is vital that we approach the issue of eating and drinking in labour in a balanced way, whether it is the evidence, the physiology, the psychology, the history or the impact on the childbearing process we are considering. With this in mind we have invited authors from different backgrounds, including consumers of maternity care, to contribute to this book.

Impact of current research

Midwives offer care to all childbearing women, regardless of actual complications or potential problems, yet the literature and research available about eating and drinking in labour has been undertaken almost exclusively by our medical colleagues. This is no surprise, as research has had a high profile on the medical agenda for longer than it has on the midwifery one. However, it means that as practising midwives we are currently making decisions about the midwifery care of women using information analysed and disseminated by medical practitioners. This situation has produced a body of 'scientific' evidence which supports the restriction of food and drink for labouring women and in doing so purports to inform practice protocols that guide midwifery practice and limit women's choice. As evidence based practice is now a priority, we are in a situation of having to demonstrate that eating and drinking in labour is safe practice if we are to re-introduce it to the midwifery care of childbearing women, when it was never confirmed to be an effective measure to reduce Mendelson's syndrome (acid aspiration) in the first place.

The other important implication of the prevalence of medical research is that there are fundamental gaps in our knowledge regarding restriction of eating and drinking in labour. Namely, the physiological impact on the labour itself, implications for the post partum healing process and the neonate, and the psychological issues. These areas are important to midwives and to childbearing women but may not have been brought to the attention or have the same research status for medical practitioners. Midwives and consumers are beginning to address the issues highlighted, with reviews of current literature (Baker, 1996; Pengelley and Gyte, 1996; Sharp, 1997) and with research and audit addressing some of the deficiencies in our knowledge (Berry, 1997; Newton and Champion, 1997; Riches, 1996; Yiannousiz, 1994).

The Confidential Enquiry into Maternal Mortality reports have included fatal cases of Mendelson's syndrome and are often critical of the practice of medical practitioners, particularly anaesthetists. This is because the incidence of Mendelson's syndrome in childbearing women is almost exclusively related to situations where women lose control of their airway, which occurs mainly during the administration of general anaesthesia. This has three implications, one being that maternity departments should be staffed with senior anaesthetic practitioners. The second is that strict protocols, which include the application of cricoid pressure during the induction of general anaesthetic, should be used for all women, from the first trimester of pregnancy to at least 48 hours post partum. The third implication is that, because it tends to be medical/anaesthetic practitioners and not midwives who are criticized, then midwives should be making significant contributions to the policies and decision-making which surround the care of *all* labouring women.

It is questionable whether greater consultation between practitioners such as doctors and midwives, who may approach the care of childbearing women with differing philosophies, is going to achieve a policy that accounts for the majority of women experiencing childbirth with no general anaesthesia. Because Mendelson's syndrome or acid aspiration is a condition associated with administration of general anaesthetic, the discussions should centre around reducing the use of general anaesthesia in parturition, as well as restricting food and drink to labouring women.

Policies and protocols

There is a perception that the autonomy of the midwife has been curtailed by the introduction of policies that limit women from eating and drinking in labour. Knowledge of a pathological condition (Mendelson's syndrome) has been applied to an event (birth) which for the majority of women is physiological. This is medicalization of midwifery practice. The application of the ethical concept of utilitarianism or 'the greatest good for the greatest number' to this issue actually conflicts with the rules and code of practice for midwives (UKCC, 1998), which takes a very different, individualized approach. Midwives are in a difficult position when a woman requests food or drink and a protocol restricts this without giving evidence. The feelings of various practitioners in the maternity setting with regard to this restriction are strong as this issue affects women's choice, midwives' practice, has implications for maternal morbidity and mortality and embodies the medicalization of childbirth.

The *Midwives Rules and Code of Practice* (UKCC, 1998) states that midwives are responsible for the care of pregnant women who fall into the category of being normal. This is upheld by the objective recommended by *Changing Childbirth* (Department of Health, 1993) of the midwife being the lead professional for at least 30% of women. This also implies that the midwife should be responsible for the decision-making that is a part of that overall responsibility to the woman. It is evident that in many cases midwives' practice and decision-making are driven by policies that are not formulated using a multidisciplinary approach and are usually informed by research that has a predominantly medical bias.

One of the pivotal issues for midwifery practice is how normality is defined. The definition offered by the *Concise Oxford Dictionary* is 'conforming to a standard, regular, usual or typical' (Sykes, 1989). As individual midwives our definition of normal hinges on our fundamental view of childbearing.

Do we see it as a physiological / emotional / social event or, do we see it as a potentially pathological event which can only be declared normal after birth, when it has been deemed to conform to the criteria by which we currently define normality. So, a normal delivery might be that which displays certain occurrences, which generally happen, for example, a spontaneous vaginal delivery, a healthy baby, a minimal blood loss, spontaneous delivery of the placenta?

What about artificial rupture of the membranes (ARM)? In a unit where there is a policy dictating ARM at 3 cm dilatation for all women, ARM would conform to the definition of normal; a regular, usual or typical event. Yet as midwives we want to protest; it is not normal, but it may be a 'typical birth'. The word which springs to mind as a replacement is 'natural'. As midwives we observe that women who labour spontaneously without the restriction of a policy often eat and drink, and so for us it would seem normal or natural to encourage women to do so. This is perhaps not the right place to begin a debate on what is normality, mainly because there is no definite answer. Substituting the word natural has political implications, not least because the whole of health care philosophy in this country could be perceived as a battle against nature, and this applies to maternity care too.

In a maternity unit where the normal practice is to restrict oral intake, a policy / guideline which liberalizes it gives midwives the support they need to practise in a physiological way. In the long term it serves to re-balance the care of normal labouring women, normalizing eating and drinking in labour so that it becomes usual practice. There may come a time when such a guideline is no longer required and policy-making then becomes a way of changing practice.

The Audit Commission (1997) looking at maternity services encourages the development of clinical guidelines and protocols. There is a feeling that policies that address emergency issues such as shoulder dystocia and postpartum haemorrhage should be formulated proactively, and implemented before a disastrous event occurs rather than in response to it (Advanced Life Support in Obstetrics, 1996). Policies should be evidence based and practitioners should be familiar with their content and practised in their procedures. It may be that some situations could be served by national guidelines for practice, a way of approaching risk management by standardizing care patterns. The previous statement reveals a question; is there a difference between protocols that deal with emergency and patently abnormal situations and those that address normal practice? We feel there is, and this is illustrated by looking at the issue of the birth environment.

Anecdotally there appears to be an inequity of care between the home and hospital environment. It seems that as we move out of the policy-driven environment of the hospital towards the home so the policy seems to lose its power over us. For instance, if we were to produce a national policy stating that no woman was allowed to eat or drink in labour at home there would be a public outcry and we would be accused of violating the human right to privacy. Yet, it is acceptable to do exactly that in hospital. For example, one of the authors' initial interest in the effects of restricting food and drink in labour was realized after reflecting on her own practice. A woman in early labour was hungry but the hospital custom and practice was to deny anything other than water (there was no policy at the time). The midwife closed the door, added the 'Do not disturb' sign and shared her sandwiches with the woman. It felt like a deception of the system, but also common sense being applied by an autonomous practitioner to a woman in 'Normal labour'. This conflict grew into the hospital's development of a more liberal guideline.

In the community setting for maternity care, policies tend to be more liberal, less in number and more geared towards handling emergency or abnormal situations. Such guidelines tend to be produced by the practitioners involved in using them. In an area in the Midlands where hospital and community trusts are separate, the policy for managing a retained placenta is different. The hospital policy states that the doctor should be called if the placenta is not delivered within 20 minutes of delivery of the baby. In the community the time limit is one hour. This is evidence of inequity of care dependent on the environment.

The making of policy in the community tends to be done by practitioners to whom the policy is appropriate. In a hospital setting it tends to be done by a multidisciplinary team, some of whom do not practise within the realms of the policy, especially if it is about normal practice. This situation results in compromise within the policy so that it pleases all members and thus hospital based maternity care is compromised and midwifery care is medicalized.

How then could this dilemma be resolved around the issue of eating and drinking in labour? There should be a team of practitioners who acknowledge each other as experts in their own field, whose sphere of practice is relevant to the issue and who are equal in terms of numbers. It is of little value having an overpowering number of midwives or doctors in a team because of the compromise that will occur. This team should also have the option to call in experts such as dieticians to fully inform their decision-making. An example team for the subject under discussion might be a midwife, an obstetrician and an anaesthetist, aided by a dietician and a physiologist who then disseminate their thoughts and draft policies among their colleagues for comment.

During this introduction several issues have been identified which are significant in the development of midwifery care. To the question of whether eating and drinking in labour is safe practice there is no straightforward answer. Current research evidence is not conclusive and it may be that trying to find a definite answer is the wrong direction in which to proceed. As carers in a maternity setting we are striving to provide women with choice, and to do that we need knowledge and the flexibility of thought to apply it to individual women.

Another issue is that of the prevalence of medical research. There is now educational and financial support for midwives to proceed with research in their chosen areas and we need to go for it! If we can collaborate with our colleagues to illuminate areas of practice that need research so much the better. As midwives we can not only use but also initiate research to redress this balance in many areas of practice.

The final issue is perhaps the most complex of all; the debate about the impact of policy on practice in the maternity setting. This debate occurs within the political arena of the National Health Service, and involves issues such as insurance cover for hospital trusts, education of all types of students and clinical practice. Midwives do not work in isolation from other practitioners and the interface we have with our medical colleagues in particular is crucial to achieving our goal of best practice. We need to move towards multidisciplinary policy-making, which accounts for the autonomy of all practitioners and applies to appropriate areas of practice.

It is because of these issues that we have come to a somewhat philosophical conclusion in this book. There are no certain answers to the questions we have asked but as practitioners – midwifery and medical – in the maternity setting we all have the same goal: to see the women and babies we care for reach the best possible outcomes. We can only achieve this by working together in policy-making and research and by acknowledging that we are all equal players in the game.

References

Advanced Life Support in Obstetrics (ALSO) (1996) *Course Syllabus*, 3rd edition. Missouri: American Academy of Family Physicians

Audit Commission (1997) *First Class Delivery: Improving Maternity Services in England and Wales*. Abingdon: Audit Commission

Baker, C. (1996) Nutrition and hydration in labour. *British Journal of Midwifery* 4 (11): 568–72

Berry, H. (1997) Feast or famine? Oral intake during labour: current evidence and practice. *British Journal of Midwifery* 5 (7): 413–17

Department of Health (1993) *Changing Childbirth Part One.* Report of the Expert Maternity Group. London: HMSO

Newton, C. and Champion, P. (1997) Oral intake in labour: Nottingham's policy formulated and audited. *British Journal of Midwifery* 5 (7): 418–22

Pengelley, L. and Gyte, G. (1996) *Eating and Drinking in Labour.* NCT evidence based briefing no 1. London: National Childbirth Trust

Riches, L. (1996) A Comparative Study on the Effects of Eating and Drinking versus a Restricted Intake during Labour. Unpublished MSc Thesis, University of Surrey Library/Royal College of Midwives Library, London

Sharp, D.A. (1997) Restriction of oral intake for women in labour. *British Journal of Midwifery* 5 (7): 408–12

Sykes, J.B. (1989) *The Concise Oxford Dictionary*, 7th edition. Oxford: Oxford University Press

United Kingdom Central Council (UKCC) (1998) *Midwives Rules and Code of Practice.* London: UKCC

Yiannousiz, K. (1994) Randomised controlled trial measuring the effects on labour of offering a light low fat diet (Abstract). *MIRIAD*, pp. 196–8 (Cheshire: Books for Midwives Press)

CHAPTER TWO

Cultural and historical perspectives on eating and drinking in labour

Carol McCormick and Penny Champion

- Alcohol, herbal concoctions, raw eggs, tea made from human hair and gunpowder have been used in labour
- Food is a culturally important substance
- Following the publication of papers by Mendelson and Parker, advice for labouring women changed in the Western world
- The usefulness of routine antacid therapy is still under question, as it does not seem to afford the protection that was anticipated
- Good perioperative care is the safest option

If we broaden our knowledge horizons about eating and drinking in labour, and look down cultural and historical avenues, it provides us with space to evaluate whether our 'Western' practices are valid. 'Without this approach, our beliefs and behaviours ... remain unexamined, since they appear to us to be "normal", "natural" and "reasonable"' (Laderman, 1988: 86). The literature which explores the issue of eating and drinking in labour through anthropological and cultural perspectives is very limited.

The culture of food

Food is a culturally important substance. It has connections with both physical and psychological well-being. 'Eat, drink and be merry' is a phrase which will be familiar, but it highlights the psychological abilities and attributes of food. If we think of a 'good night out' it will more often than not include food and drink. Equally, food is considered to be a provider of strength and special food substances are used to procure good health. The growing market in vitamin supplements, magazines about healthy eating and an increasing public awareness of the health promoting and damaging properties of certain foods, demonstrates the cultural importance of food in our society. Food in its many forms is considered to be a life force.

It seems strange that this significant substance which sustains life should be restricted during the time of childbearing – a time when physical and psychological strength are required.

Anthropological work in the field of birth practices (Laderman, 1988: 86–7) highlights the importance of considering the 'custom' of restricting eating and drinking in labour within the context of the society as a whole. There are many factors which impose upon women's activity in labour and these include the role of the medical profession, the role of the midwife, the position of the woman within the team of carers and the relative power of all these people in the childbearing process.

The same author highlights areas where Western attitudes to childbearing differ from those of Malay women. The first is the autonomy of the woman within the team of carers. Western women are often divested of their autonomy, with the obstetrician and midwife taking lead roles in the woman's care. This is in contrast to the experience of the Malay woman, who considers herself the centre of the process with the knowledgeable midwife to assist her. This point was made before the publication of *Changing Childbirth* (Department of

Health, 1993) and emphasizes the importance of women-centred care and the impact it can have on outcome.

Laderman (1988: 87) also makes reference to the effect that maternal mortality and morbidity has upon our practice. The triennial Confidential Enquiry into Maternal Deaths (Department of Health, 1975 to 1998) includes in each edition a number of women who have died because of aspiration of gastric contents (Mendelson's syndrome). In our quest to prevent these deaths, midwives and obstetricians impose restrictions on eating and drinking in labour in the hope that women will have as near as possible 'empty' stomachs and will not aspirate their gastric contents during general anaesthesia. The goal is an admirable one but we have become aware that the practice does not achieve what we wish it to. Laderman criticizes our pathological view of childbirth, which is fuelled by reports such as the Confidential Enquiry. This pathological view imposes restrictions on all women, 'sacrificing the comfort of many in order to (possibly) preclude the death of a few' (Laderman, 1988: 87). This point is also raised by Cram Elsberry (1990: 242), when she estimates that the incidence of death from aspiration pneumonitis in the United States in 1986 was 2.6 per million live births. The 'perils' of childbirth are allowed to override the woman's needs in labour, and to erode her control over the process. Equally, they also erode the autonomy of obstetricians and midwives in providing physiological care.

Broach and Newton (1988: 81–5), in their findings related to historical and cultural practices around eating and drinking in labour, reveal an amazing diversity. Although they found that historical records of the practices surrounding diet for women in normal labour were scarce because childbirth tended to be a family affair, they note that food and beverages have been used during labour as nourishment and medicine. In many cases food and beverages were given as 'treatments' to ease pain, to hasten labour, to strengthen uterine contractions and to promote relaxation. These foods varied from culture to culture and included alcohol, herbal concoctions, raw eggs, tea made from human hair and gunpowder. Some cultures restricted any oral substance to be taken during labour, fearing the effect it may have.

Texts relating to American practice (DeLee, 1904: 104–5) indicate that food and drink was positively encouraged to preserve the woman's strength, and that drinks especially should be given even if the woman vomits. So, it would seem that in the vast majority of cultures and up until the 1940s, women were encouraged to eat and drink in order to sustain themselves during childbirth, and indeed in order to prevent complications such as prolonged labour occurring (DeLee, 1904: 104–5).

The 1940s saw the beginning of the use of general anaesthesia during the childbearing process (Ludka and Roberts, 1993: 199). Many women were anaesthetized during the second stage of labour as a routine practice (Broach and Newton, 1988: 82). It was also at this time that medical practitioners began to suspect that the process of labour may have a delaying effect on gastric emptying, although the research done at that time presented a confusing picture with many different measurement methods being used and no firm conclusions being reached (Wilson, 1978: 54). These two factors, combined with an increasing interest in the causes of maternal morbidity/mortality and the increase in hospital/institutional confinement which began in the early 1950s (Oakley, 1986: 215), prompted medical practitioners such as Mendelson (1946: 191–205) and Parker (1956: 16–19) to study the aspiration of gastric contents in childbearing women.

The history of Mendelson's syndrome

Mendelson (1946: 191) undertook a huge retrospective study of 44 016 pregnancies of women who attended the New York Lying-in Hospital from 1932 to1945. The incidence of aspiration of stomach contents was 0.15% (66 women). The women who suffered from aspiration had a slightly higher incidence of prolonged labour (30 hours or more) and the delivery details reveal a spontaneous delivery rate of only 44%, a caesarean section rate of 21% and an instrumental delivery rate of 35%. Slightly more than half of them had operative intervention which required longer administration and greater depth of general anaesthesia, than those delivering spontaneously. The delivery details state that all the women who aspirated were anaesthetized to some degree during the second stage of labour. The anaesthetic used was a mixture of gas, oxygen and ether.

Mendelson does not clarify in his article the routine practices in the hospital, such as whether all women were anaesthetized for the second stage of labour and whether women ate and drank in labour. It is also unclear whether the total number of women fell into a high-risk group, which might be suspected if they were attending hospital for delivery at that time.

During the study period there were 66 recorded cases of aspiration of stomach contents into the lungs. This finding in itself could arouse suspicion because 'regurgitation may not easily be recognized' (Parker, 1954: 65), and because cases of aspiration asphyxia are only confirmed on post mortem. In Mendelson's study, the type of material aspirated was recorded in 45 cases. Two women died of suffocation because their tracheas became blocked with solid material; the remaining three who aspirated solid material managed to cough up the obstruction. The other 40 women aspirated liquid material and developed an asthma-like syndrome known as aspiration pneumonitis. All these women recovered, despite some being critically ill. It is not known whether the women included in this study ate or drank during labour, or what method of anaesthesia was used in their care.

Despite the imperfections of his work, Mendelson's paper has had a very significant impact upon current midwifery, anaesthetic and obstetric care.

In 1956, Parker published a paper that analysed the mortality of women in the Birmingham area from aspiration asphyxia. He recorded 8 deaths due largely or entirely to aspiration asphyxia, which amounted to a mortality rate of 1 in 27 000 births in the City of Birmingham area. All the case histories given by Parker are of women who would be considered high risk by current standards. No reference is made to whether the woman had eaten or drunk during labour. The use of anaesthesia for delivery is mentioned by Parker. He notes that where instrumental deliveries were performed at home, with ether or chloroform, there was no incidence of aspiration of gastric contents. In the same time period, a smaller number of women had instrumental delivery in hospital and four died from aspiration asphyxia. It is possible from the description of the case histories to suppose that this group of women had general anaesthesia. Parker states that important factors in preventing anaesthetic-related deaths are: skilled, readily available anaesthetists, use of local analgesia wherever possible, maternal position at the time of anaesthesia and of delivery, and the use of cuffed endotracheal tubes. These recommendations are remarkably similar to those made by the Confidential Enquiry reports.

Parker's work (1954: 65) prompted much correspondence in the medical literature and was discussed at length at the Royal Society of Medicine in 1955 (Crawford, 1956: 201). Action was required and anaesthetists took on the role of improving practice because of the exclusive relationship between aspiration of gastric contents and general anaesthesia. Crawford (1956: 201) published a series of articles in the *British Journal of Anaesthesia*. He addressed many issues pertaining to the anaesthetic care of childbearing women, including the drugs and techniques used for inducing anaesthesia, and the issue of vomiting.

He reminds us that it was generally accepted that, during labour, gastric emptying time was prolonged. 'If this is so, then there are two prophylactic measures which may be taken to prevent vomiting. Firstly, women in labour may be starved; secondly, a diet may be given which will be easily aspirated [via a tube] should an anaesthetic be needed'. Crawford was not keen to starve women in labour; he had already tried it, and found women who had been starved in labour recalled their hunger as a very unpleasant memory. Instead, a semi-fluid diet was introduced which resulted in minimal vomiting and minimal use of the stomach tube to aspirate the gastric contents prior to anaesthesia. This led Crawford to recommend that labouring women should be given a semi-solid/fluid diet in labour which he found was not only easy to aspirate should the need arise but was also rapidly digested.

It is interesting to note that ten years after the publication of Mendelson's paper in 1946, neither Parker (1956: 16–19) nor Crawford (1956: 201–8) refer to the aspiration of gastric contents as Mendelson's syndrome, and Mendelson's paper does not seem to have had the immediate effect on practice that we might assume. It would appear from a comment made by Crawford (1986: 920) that the paper published by Parker (1956: 16–19) had more influence on British practice than Mendelson's work: *'Is it not intriguing that, in England and Wales, the number of maternal deaths from acid aspiration apparently rose only after the appearance of Parker's 1956 paper led to severe dietary restriction in labour, amounting in most units to almost starvation?'* Even more interesting was that Parker made no recommendations about dietary restriction during labour in his 1956 paper.

Following the publication of Mendelson's (1946) and Parker's (1956) papers, advice to doctors and midwives caring for labouring women began to change. The risks of vomiting during anaesthesia were recognized and it was assumed that eating and drinking in labour increased the risk of vomiting (DeLee, 1947: 237). Various obstetric and anaesthetic textbooks (Mayes, 1953: 272; Hingson and Hellman, 1956: 111; McLennan, 1962: 163; Philipp, 1962: 141; Masani, 1964: 141–3;

Townsend, 1964: 123) recommended different dietary strategies for reducing aspiration asphyxia. These ranged from complete abstinence from eating and drinking, to a light diet in early labour, drinking only, and taking easily digestible solids. There was no consensus of opinion about what was the best method. However, the recommendation to withhold solid foods in particular persists as part of a package of preventative measures to this day (Smith and Bogod, 1995).

Interestingly, a midwifery text written by an obstetrician from 1972 suggests that women should eat and drink in labour: 'fluids such as water and tea are necessary and food should be sieved' (Hallum, 1972: 65). By 1980, Towler and Butler-Manuel (p. 318) were suggesting that 'normal women in very early labour should eat something light and easily digestible' but that formal meals should not be given. They positively encourage the addition of glucose powder to any drinks the woman takes. They also introduce the idea of assessing the risk for general anaesthesia before considering feeding a labouring woman. In 1988, *Maye's Midwifery* (Sweet, 1988: 189) suggests that food should be withheld completely and fluids restricted to sips of water or ice chips. More recent midwifery texts (Henderson, 1997; Sweet, 1997) cautiously encourage oral intake. Advice for practitioners in maternity care seems very conflicting.

The condition which Mendelson observed in his work is now generally referred to as acid aspiration syndrome (Sharp, 1997). Crawford (1984) describes the syndrome as follows. Following aspiration of acidic material, the respiratory epithelium and vascular endothelium are damaged, leading to leakage of protein rich fluid into the alveoli and interstitial spaces. Subsequently necrotic changes occur in the affected regions of the lungs, accompanied by sloughing of the mucosa, which provides potential sites for infection. The immediate response is bronchospasm which might be localized or become generalized, shortly succeeded by reduced perfusion. Hypoxaemia and severe metabolic acidosis result.

Death may result from large food particles inhaled into the lungs or from pneumonitis due to aspiration of acid or small food particles (Mendelson, 1946).

The influence of the reports on the Confidential Enquiry into Maternal Deaths

This document, published triennially by the Department of Health, is an audit of all maternal deaths occurring in England and Wales (and throughout the United Kingdom since 1985). Expert practitioners review the cases and in the light of research evidence provide recommendations for practice.

An overview of the comments and recommendations which appear at the end of each chapter about deaths associated with anaesthesia, from 1970 to the present, reveal how influential this document is, and how it appears to have affected practice relating to the care of women who were at risk of aspirating stomach contents.

Recommendations

Skilled staff

One of the recurring themes has been the recommendation that skilled and senior anaesthetists and experienced help be on hand at all times wherever there are childbearing women who may need general anaesthesia. Childbearing women are recognized as being particularly vulnerable to the effects of aspiration of gastric contents, although the reasons for this are not wholly evident. Because of the centralization of maternity provision over the same period it is now feasible to expect every labour ward area to have a consultant anaesthetist on the premises or very near by at all times.

Cricoid pressure

In the early 1970s the application of cricoid pressure was not routine when intubating pregnant women who required general anaesthesia. Since 1973 it has been mentioned in every report with detailed instructions appearing in two of the reports about how to apply cricoid pressure correctly. It is currently accepted practice that every pregnant woman who requires a general anaesthetic should be treated as a 'crash' intubation (i.e. assuming she has a full stomach), the procedure for which includes cricoid pressure.

Antacid therapy

The 1973–75 report (Department of Health, 1979) revealed that antacid prophylaxis was a routine procedure but that its effectiveness in protecting against Mendelson's syndrome needed to be re-examined in light of the fact that all the women who died following aspiration of stomach contents had had adequate antacid therapy. The report also suggested that antacid therapy be considered as part of a 'package' of preventative measures. It is not clear from the report what substance was used as an antacid at that time but it was probably Mist.Mag.Trisil. B.P.C. (Scott, 1978: 48). The 1979–81 report (Department of Health, 1986) revealed that particulate antacids such as Mist.Mag.Trisil B.P.C. could be as damaging to lung tissue as acid stomach contents, and also that the volume of the stomach contents was increased by giving this mixture. H_2-receptor antagonists (ranitidine) were recommended for the first time as a way of reducing gastric acidity and continued to be recommended in all following reports. The use of sodium citrate as a non-particulate antacid was mentioned in the 1982–84 report (Department of Health, 1989), with the implication that, along with the use of H_2-receptor antagonists, it could be administered in a small volume prior to intubation thus preventing the increase in volume of stomach contents. Since 1984 the use of non-particulate antacid mixtures has become common practice prior to intubation, although the effectiveness of antacid therapy in protecting against Mendelson's syndrome was again questioned when the one woman who died was found to have had full antacid prophylaxis, including administration of intravenous ranitidine.

Reducing the volume of stomach contents

The 1979–81 report (Department of Health, 1986) stated very clearly that no food or fluid should be given by mouth in labour. This comment was not discriminatory in any way: no labouring woman was exempted from it. This recommendation has not been made since that report.

This same report also drew attention to the effect of narcotic analgesia on gastric emptying. Although research work was inconclusive with respect to the effect of labour on stomach emptying, it was evident that narcotic analgesia such as pethidine and diamorphine slowed gastric emptying appreciably and added to the risk of aspiration. In fact in all subsequent reports it has been recommended that for women known to have had narcotic analgesia, consideration should be given to emptying their stomachs via a nasogastric tube prior to intubation.

Postoperative care

The 1988–90 report (Department of Health, 1994) highlighted the importance of good postoperative care, and recommended that midwifery staff who 'recover' women following general anaesthetic should be specifically trained in monitoring, care of the airway and resuscitative procedures and should be supervised by a defined anaesthetist at all times.

It is evident from the recommendations made by the Confidential Enquiry that the majority of changes have centred around anaesthetic practice. Improvements in the experience of staff and the techniques used at intubation have had a big impact upon the maternal mortality associated with aspiration of gastric contents.

The usefulness of current regimes of antacid therapy are still under question, as it does not seem to afford the protection which is anticipated.

The delay in gastric emptying associated with narcotic analgesia is well documented and midwives as well as anaesthetists should heed this when caring for labouring women. All three women who died because of aspiration of gastric contents in the 1985–87 and 1988–90 reports (Department of Health, 1991, 1994) had had narcotic analgesia in labour.

Table 2.1 reveals how the incidence of death following aspiration of stomach contents has lessened considerably over the period since 1973. The reasons for this are probably related not only to changes in practice around care of women requiring general anaesthesia but also to factors such as the increasing use of regional anaesthesia for operative procedures, which means that women can protect their own airway, and the reduction in the use of narcotic analgesia, which is known to increase the emptying time of the stomach (Nimmo, 1975a: 890; Nimmo, 1975b: 509; Wilson, 1978: 59).

Table 2.1 Numbers of maternal deaths attributable to aspiration of gastric contents

Year	Total number of maternities	Total maternal deaths known to Enquiry	Number of deaths attributed to aspiration of stomach contents
1973–1975	1 921 568	390	13
1976–1978	1 748 851	325	11
1979–1981	1 923 725	268	8
1982–1984	1 888 753	209	7
1985–1987	2 268 766	223	1
1988–1990	2 360 309	238	2
1991–1993	2 315 204	228	1
1994–1996	2 197 640	268	0

Source: Report on Confidential Enquiries into Maternal Deaths in the United Kingdom (Department of Health, triennial, 1975–98; England and Wales only to 1985)

The history of starving women in labour

There have been two surveys of practices in maternity units in England and Wales, Garcia and Garforth (1989: 155–62) and Michael *et al.* (1991: 1071–3). Although not directly comparable because of their differing samples and questions both surveys revealed a wide variation in practices surrounding feeding in labour in consultant units. In a highly informative document, Pengelley and Gyte (1996: 4) have summarized the findings of these two surveys (see Table 2.2). It would seem from these findings that practice became less liberal in the five years between these surveys, and inconsistency in opinion is clearly visible.

Table 2.2 Policies for eating and drinking in labour

Recommendations	1984	1989
No food at all in labour	39%	68.3%
No food in established labour	39%	31.7%
Nothing prescribed orally	2%	3.6%
Sips of water and ice cubes only	98%	94.6%
Drinks other than water	67%	44%

Source: Pengelley and Gyte, 1996

It is impossible to know the range of practices relating to oral intake in labour throughout the country. It would appear that the home environment offers women more choice about eating and drinking. Cram Elsberry (1990: 243), in a survey of 86 American women who were attending hospital for delivery, found that they had all eaten in the 8 hours prior to admission and the majority were admitted in active labour. This finding is reflected by the audit in Nottingham (Newton and Champion, 1997: 421), where 75% of the sample ate during labour, 51.8% (128) whilst at home. Interestingly, the majority of the women in Nottingham had been advised to eat when they went into labour by their community midwife whereas the American women had very little advice given to them. In England the culture of starving women who come into hospital in labour persists and this may be why community midwives advise women to 'stock up' before they come in. That women eat in early labour may reveal that they are more comfortable eating at home, in a familiar environment, and able to eat and drink the foodstuffs they choose. It may also indicate a physiological need for oral intake in early labour. The other more political factor is that whilst women remain in their own homes, those policies which guide hospital practice are irrelevant, as midwives, obstetricians and anaesthetists we have no power to impose a restriction on oral intake.

Since 1989 a review of the literature reveals an increasing number of articles written by midwives about oral intake in labour. What is it in the current climate that has led to the practice of restricting oral intake in labour being questioned?

The Winterton Report (House of Commons Health Committee, 1991: xciv) and *Changing Childbirth* (Department of Health, 1993: 5) both called for women to have control and choice in the care they receive during childbearing. At the same time, information resources such as the publication *Effective Care in Pregnancy and Childbirth* (Chalmers *et al.*, 1989) and the Cochrane Library have promoted the concept of evidence based practice. It is impossible to help women reach informed decisions about their care unless we have information to impart to them. In the case of oral intake in labour, the evidence does not appear to support the activity, as mentioned in other chapters of this book. In consequence, there is increasing interest in liberalizing policies about oral intake in labour, many of which are being prompted by midwives (Yiannousiz, 1994; Baker, 1996; Riches, 1996; Newton and Champion, 1997).

Conclusion

The cultural and historical influences mentioned above have had a significant impact on the practice of eating and drinking in labour. Food was considered an important substance for sustaining women in labour, not only nutritionally but also psychologically. It was 'normal' for labouring women to eat and drink if they wanted to. The advent of hospitalized birth, anaesthetics in the birth process and research into the consequences of these practices have put a question mark over the issue of oral intake in labour. It must be acknowledged that all these influences have had profoundly positive effects upon the safety of birth, but they have also undermined the confidence of women and practitioners in trusting women's instincts and knowledge about how to give birth successfully. How can we as midwives (obstetricians and anaesthetists) claim to know what is best for every woman we care for. We have very little research that we can generalize to every woman and this is emphasized by Odent (1994): 'we still have to accept that a woman's nutritional needs during labour are too complex to be managed by a birth attendant'. Preventing women from eating and drinking in labour is an intervention, but so is making women eat and drink. We do not want to replace one restrictive policy with another. The key issue is, what does the woman want to do?

References

Baker, C. (1996) Nutrition and hydration in labour. *British Journal of Midwifery* 4 (11): 568–72

Broach, J. and Newton, N. (1988) Food and beverages in Labor. Part 1: Cross-cultural and historical practices. *Birth*, 15 (2): 81–5

Chalmers, I. *et al.* (1989) *Effective Care in Pregnancy and Childbirth*. Oxford: Oxford University Press

Cram Elsberry, C. (1990) Nutrition in labor. In: *A Midwife's Gift: Love, Skill and Knowledge*. Proceedings of the ICM 22nd International Congress, 7–12 October 1990, Kobe, Japan. Tokyo: ICM, pp. 241–3

Crawford, J.S. (1956) Some aspects of obstetric anaesthesia. *British Journal of Anaesthesia* 28: 146–54, 201–7

Crawford, J.S. (1984) *Principles and Practice of Obstetric Anaesthesia*. Oxford: Blackwell Sciences, pp. 269–84

Crawford, J.S. (1986) Maternal mortality from Mendelson's syndrome. *Lancet* i (19 April): 587

DeLee, J.B. (1904) *Notes on Obstetrics*. Chicago: Kenfield, pp. 104–5

DeLee, J.B. and Greenhill, J.P. (1947) *Principles and Practice of Obstetrics*, 9th edition. Philadelphia: Saunders, p. 237

Department of Health (1975) *Report on Confidential Enquiries into Maternal Deaths in England and Wales, 1970–72*, edited by H Arthure *et al*. London: HMSO

Department of Health (1979) *Report on Confidential Enquiries into Maternal Deaths in England and Wales, 1973–75*, edited by J.S. Tomkinson *et al*. London: HMSO

Department of Health (1982) *Report on Confidential Enquiries into Maternal Deaths in England and Wales, 1976–79*, edited by J.S. Tomkinson *et al*. London: HMSO

Department of Health (1986) *Report on Confidential Enquiries into Maternal Deaths in England and Wales, 1979–81*, edited by A. Turnbull *et al*. London: HMSO

Department of Health (1989) *Report on Confidential Enquiries into Maternal Deaths in England and Wales, 1982–84*, edited by A. Turnbull *et al*. London: HMSO

Department of Health (1991) *Report on Confidential Enquiries into Maternal Deaths in the United Kingdom 1985–87*. London: HMSO

Department of Health (1993) *Changing Childbirth: Part One*. Report of the Expert Maternity Group. London: HMSO

Department of Health (1994) *Report on Confidential Enquiries into Maternal Deaths in the United Kingdom, 1988–90*. London: HMSO

Department of Health (1996) *Report on Confidential Enquiries into Maternal Deaths in the United Kingdom, 1991–93*, edited by B.M. Hibbard *et al*. London: HMSO

Department of Health (1998) *Report on Confidential Enquiries into Maternal Deaths in the United Kingdom 1994–96*, edited by G. Lewis *et al*. London: HMSO

Garcia, J. and Garforth, S. (1989) Labour and delivery routines in English consultant maternity units. *Midwifery* 5: 155–62

Hallum, J.L. (1972) *Midwifery*. London: English Universities Press

Henderson, C. (ed.) (1997) *Essential Midwifery*. London: Mosby

Hingson, R.A. and Hellman, L.M. (1956) *Anaesthesia for Obstetrics*. Philadelphia: Lippincott

House of Commons Health Committee (1991) Session 1991–1992. *Second Report: Maternity Services* (The Winterton Report), Volume 1. London: HMSO

Laderman, C. (1988) Cross-cultural perspectives on birth practices. *Birth* 15 (2): 86–7

Ludka, L.M. and Roberts, C.C. (1993) Eating and drinking in labor. *Journal of Nurse-Midwifery* 38 (4): 199–207

Masani, K.M. (1964) *A Textbook of Obstetrics*. Bombay: Popular Prakashan

Mayes, B.T. (1953) *A Textbook of Obstetrics*. Sydney

McLennan, C.E. (1962) *Synopsis of Obstetrics*. St Louis: Mosby

Mendelson, C.L. (1946) The aspiration of stomach contents into the lungs during obstetric anaesthesia. *American Journal of Obstetrics and Gynecology* 52: 191–205

Michael, S. *et al.* (1991) Policies for oral intake during labour. *Anaesthesia* 46: 1017–73

Newton, C. and Champion, P. (1997) Oral intake in labour: Nottingham's policy formulated and audited. *British Journal of Midwifery* 5 (7): 418–22

Nimmo, W.S., Wilson, J. and Prescott, L.F. (1975a) Narcotic analgesics and delayed gastric emptying during labour. *The Lancet* i (19 April): 890–3

Nimmo, W.S., Heading, R.C., Wilson, J., Tothill, P. and Prescott, L.F. (1975b) Inhibition of gastric emptying and drug absorption by narcotic analgesics. *British Journal of Clinical Pharmacology* 2: (6): 509–13

Oakley, A. (1986) *The Captured Womb*. Oxford: Blackwell.

Odent, M. (1994) Labouring women are not marathon runners. *Birth* 31 (Autumn): 23–51

Parker, R.B. (1954) Risk from the aspiration of vomit during obstetric anaesthesia. *British Medical Journal* ii: 65–9

Parker, R.B. (1956) Maternal death from aspiration asphyxia. *British Medical Journal* 7 July: 16–19

Pengelley, L. and Gyte, G. (1996) *Eating and Drinking in Labour. NCT Evidence Based Briefing No. 1.* London: National Childbirth Trust

Philipp, E.E. (1962) *Obstetrics and Gynaecology*. London: HK Lewis

Riches, L. (1996) A Comparative Study on the Effects of Eating and Drinking versus a Restricted Intake during Labour. Unpublished MSc thesis, University of Surrey Library/Royal College of Midwives Library, London

Scott, D.B. (1978) History of Mendelson's syndrome. *Journal of International Medical Research* 6 (Supplement 1): 47–9

Sharp, D.A. (1997) Restriction of oral intake for women in

labour. *British Journal of Midwifery* 5 (7): 408–12

Smith, I.D.and Bogod, D.G. (1995) Feeding in labour. *Bailliere's Clinical Anaesthesiology* 9 (4): 735–47

Sweet, B. (ed.) (1988) *Maye's Midwifery: A Textbook for Midwives*. London: Bailliere Tindall

Sweet, B. (ed.) (1997) *Maye's Midwifery: A Textbook for Midwives*. London: Bailliere Tindall

Towler, J. and Butler-Manuel, R. (1980) *Modern Obstetrics for Student Midwives*. London: Lloyd-Luke

Townsend, L. (1964) *Obstetrics for Students*. New York: Cambridge University Press

Wilson, J. (1978) Gastric emptying in labour: some recent findings and their clinical significance. *Journal of International Medical Research* 6 (Supplement 1): 54–60

Yiannousiz, K. (1994) Randomized controlled trial measuring the effects on labour of offering a light, low fat diet (Abstract). *MIRIAD*, pp. 196–8 (Cheshire: Books for Midwives Press)

CHAPTER THREE

Labouring over food: the dietician's view

Ann Micklewright and Penny Champion

- Most women wish to eat and drink in early labour
- Fasting does not guarantee an empty stomach or a pH of more than 2.5
- Fluid and calorific requirements of labouring women are not known

Fasting during labour is intended to decrease or eliminate stomach contents in order to prevent vomiting or regurgitation of gastric contents into the airway during obstetric anaesthesia. A number of authors agree that there is an increased risk of maternal mortality and morbidity if gastric contents with a volume greater than 0.4 ml/kg (28 ml for a 70 kg woman) and/or with a pH of less than 2.5 are aspirated (Moir and Thornburn, 1986).

The 'pregnant' stomach

In order for acid aspiration syndrome to occur, three factors must be present. The stomach contents must be of a volume and nature to cause lung damage, the stomach contents must reflux or be vomited in order to reach the pharynx, and they must enter the lungs (Smith and Bogod, 1995).

Vomiting occurs when peristaltic waves are reversed and the contents of the stomach are propelled up the oesophagus. There are certain factors which increase the probability of vomiting in a pregnant woman and these include delayed stomach emptying, which may be caused by narcotic analgesia (Nimmo *et al.*, 1975; Holdsworth, 1978; Wilson, 1978), emotional strain and vomitable material in the stomach (Atkinson *et al.*, 1987). O'Reilly *et al.* (1993) conducted a study with 106 low-risk mothers. Given the choice, all women chose to eat and/or drink throughout all stages of labour. Of the 20 women who vomited, only eight vomited more than once and none experienced a poor outcome. This study concludes that there is little reason to routinely restrict food and drink during low-risk labour. Obviously, to a labouring woman who is fully conscious and has control of her airway, vomiting, although unpleasant, does not put her at risk of acid aspiration syndrome. In the audit by Newton and Champion (1997) there were 56 women who ate whilst labouring in hospital, out of a sample of 250. Thirty-four of these women vomited at some point during their labour and several commented that it was better to have something in your stomach even if you were sick, than be retching on an empty stomach. Work by Scrutton *et al.* (1999) paid particular attention to the volumes vomited by women who had eaten a light diet in labour. Women who ate in labour ($n = 45$) were found to be twice as likely to vomit at some point during their labour, although just under 50% of them did so after the administration of intramuscular Syntometrine. The volumes they vomited were significantly larger ($p = 0.001$) than those vomited by women who had been given water only. Both groups of women vomited volumes of more than the suggested danger volume of 0.4 ml/kg body weight and the pH of the vomit was not measured. The authors suggest that 'the presence of undigested solid food particles in the vomitus is probably of greater importance as a cause of mortality'.

Regurgitation is a more passive act which can occur with very little warning, when the pressure exerted at the lower oesophageal sphincter (LOS), situated at the junction of the oesophagus and stomach, is lower than the pressure exerted by the stomach contents. Factors which increase the likelihood of passive regurgitation during anaesthesia in a pregnant woman are: large volumes of fluid in the stomach with a pH of less than three, raised intra-abdominal pressure and relaxation of the cricopharyngeal sphincter caused by muscle relaxants (Atkinson, 1987). To prevent regurgitation of the stomach contents, it is essential to maintain a high pressure at the LOS. The hormone gastrin (produced in the mucous membrane of the pyloric stomach) and high protein foods such as lean meat, white fish and skimmed milk increase LOS pressure. Cigarette smoking and certain foods and drinks such as alcohol, fats, chocolate, regular and decaffeinated coffee, cola, peppermint, onions and garlic, reduce it (Escott-Stump, 1992). Interestingly, there is conflicting evidence about the production of the hormone gastrin in pregnancy, some suggesting that production is raised and others that it remains the same (Smith and Bogod, 1995).

The physiology of pregnancy is such that reflux appears to occur more readily, evidenced by some 80% of women reporting symptoms of 'indigestion' and 'heartburn' (Bainbridge et al., 1983). This may be because of the rise in intra-gastric pressure caused by the volume of the pregnant uterus and/or because of the reduced muscle tone at the lower oesophageal sphincter which may be a result of the effect of progesterone (Smith and Bogod, 1995).

Does fasting keep the stomach empty?

Ludka and Roberts (1993), after reviewing the literature, stated that attempting to keep the stomach empty appears to be an impossible task. Roberts and Shirley (1976) concluded a study of the gastric contents of labouring women by stating that 'no time interval between the last meal and the onset of labour guaranteed a stomach volume of less than 100 ml'. This finding has meant that all labouring women who require a general anaesthetic are considered to have a full stomach and the appropriate anaesthetic technique should be employed.

The research that has been undertaken to investigate possible delay in gastric emptying in pregnant and labouring women has not presented a clear picture (Wilson, 1978). Each study that found a delay appears to have a contradictory study which refutes that finding. Part of the problem lies with the differing methods of investigation used which make the studies incomparable. Wilson (1978) used paracetamol absorption to investigate the rate of gastric emptying in labouring women. He found that paracetamol absorption for early labour with no analgesia and postpartum women was normal. For women who were in established labour and who had received narcotic analgesia the absorption was markedly delayed. The group of women who were in established labour but had no analgesia showed some evidence of gastric delay but this was minimal compared with those women who had had narcotic analgesia. Women in established labour who had had epidural analgesia showed similar patterns to women in established labour who had had no analgesia. Wilson concludes 'it would appear that labour alone may effect a degree of delay in gastric emptying. This delay is grossly aggravated by the use of three commonly administered analgesics – diamorphine, pethidine and pentazocine'.

A small and more recent study by Carp and co-workers (1992), using ultrasound, demonstrated that 16 out of 39 parturients in active labour had food in their stomachs despite fasting for 8–24 hours.

It is interesting to note that none of the women who took part in studies relating to gastric emptying, apart from those included in the work of Carp *et al.* (1992), was assessed using normal food and fluids. It is known that the volume and nature of gastric content can affect the emptying time. The only natural stimulus to gastric emptying is gastric distension. The larger the volume of food the faster the stomach empties. Liquids empty faster than solids, which have to be broken down to particles of 1 mm in diameter before they can pass through the pyloric sphincter. Large lumps can remain in the stomach for as long as 9 hours and will continue to stimulate gastric secretion (Davenport, 1982). Large lumps of food can cause suffocation if aspirated and are as much a danger as acidic gastric contents. It is of interest that liquids empty faster when the subject is sitting or lying on the right side (Rombeau and Cauldwell, 1984). Other factors that inhibit gastric emptying are shown in Table 3.1.

Table3.1 Factors that inhibit gastric emptying

Osmolarity	Hypo- or hypertonic solutions (solutions between 5 and 10% simple sugars empty at the same rate as water)
Acid	Proportionally to the concentration of acid in the duodenum
Fats	Fatty acids with a chain length of 12–14 carbon atoms (milk and milk products) inhibit gastric emptying more than those with a chain length of 16–18 (meat products), unsaturated fats more so than saturated
Protein	Some amino acids, e.g. tryptophan
High energy foods	The higher the energy content of the food the slower the emptying, e.g. fats
Temperature	Hot and cold liquids
Drugs	Narcotic analgesia

Source: Rombeau and Cauldwell, 1984

Drugs such as metoclopramide have been used to increase gastric emptying. Research by Howard and Sharp (1973) on labouring women who were given metoclopramide showed a significant improvement in gastric emptying. The effect upon the gastric emptying times for women who have had pethidine has also been studied (Murphy *et al.*, 1984) and again a significant improvement was noted, although normal rates of gastric emptying were not restored by the administration of metoclopramide.

Does fasting affect gastric content pH?

The major stimulus to acid secretion is ingestion of food and/or drink. When food enters the stomach, gastric distension and the release of gastrin stimulate the gastric glands to secrete gastric juice, which contains hydrochloric acid. Once a pH of 1.5 is reached gastrin is inactivated and further acid production ceases. Basal or fasting acid secretion varies over time and is usually about 5–10% of the maximum rate. The highest output is in the early morning and the lowest in late evening. (This may have implications for high-risk mothers delivering in the early morning hours.) Basal output is probably due to spontaneous release of gastrin or vagal nerve stimulation. Acid secretion continues despite the absence of food. Roberts and Shirley (1976) highlighted that four out of six women whose last meal was more than 20 hours prior to delivery had an aspirate with a pH below 1.8. It cannot be assumed that fasting will result in gastric contents with a pH greater than 2.5. Hester and Heath (1977) also found 'high volumes of acid gastric juice even after prolonged starvation'.

Amino acids and partially digested protein stimulate the secretion of gastrin whilst carbohydrate and fat have no effect (Richardson *et al.*, 1976). Caffeine and alcohol increase acid directly without stimulating gastrin secretion. Large quantities of milk first buffer then stimulate acidity (Escott-Stump, 1992). Hypertonic glucose solutions (>10%) taken orally or given intravenously suppress acid secretion. Providing the labouring mother with hypertonic drinks may seem a useful approach but unfortunately hypertonic drinks also inhibit gastric emptying. Health professionals and pregnant women should be made aware of this during their education about care in labour. Fasting does not ensure that the gastric contents are less acidic. What is interesting, however, is the observation that when food is ingested the pH of the gastric content rises (Lewis, 1991).

What are the physiological consequences of restricting food and fluid intake?

During any period of fasting the body's priority is to meet its needs for energy. It will do this by generating energy from reserves of protein, fat and carbohydrate.

Carbohydrate is stored as glycogen in the liver and muscles. Glycogen is a complex molecule composed of many thousands of glucose units whose structure permits the rapid release of glucose for use as energy. The energy potential of stored liver glycogen is around 3.4 MJ (800 kcal), that of muscle glycogen 8.4 MJ (2000 kcal). These estimates apply to the non-pregnant woman; there is no literature to support any change in pregnancy.

Body fat stores represent a much greater energy reserve. For example, a slim woman weighing 60 kg at the start of pregnancy will be carrying about 12 kg of storage fat (Hill, 1992), which has an energy potential of around 360 MJ (90 000kcal). By full term this storage fat will have increased by 2–4 kg to provide an energy reserve for lactation (COMA (A), 1991).

The estimated energy requirement for a pregnant woman at term is 8.9 MJ (2140 kcal/day) (COMA (B), 1991). By simple arithmetic, the pregnant woman should have sufficient energy within her body fat stores to last for 42 days of fasting, therefore a short fast during labour should cause few problems. However, the body's response to fasting, even in normal circumstances, is not so straightforward.

At the beginning of a fast, glucose from glycogen stores and fatty acids from body fat stores begin to flow into the cells, where through a series of chemical reactions they are broken down to provide energy. Within 48–72 hours glycogen stores are depleted and most cells become dependent on fatty acids for their fuel. Brain and nerve cells are the exception and require glucose for fuel. New glucose is obtained by deamination of amino acids released from muscle protein. During the first few days of a fast, body protein will provide 90% of this glucose, but as the fast continues brain cells and some nervous tissues gradually adapt to utilize an alternative energy source – the ketone body, which is formed in the liver from the incomplete oxidation of fatty acids. Small amounts of ketone bodies are a normal part of the blood biochemistry. When the concentration of ketone bodies rises, they spill over into the urine taking large quantities of sodium and potassium with them, which may cause a decrease in the pH of the blood, resulting in dehydration.

The response to fasting during late pregnancy seems to be accelerated (Felig *et al.*, 1972). These authors noted the appearance of ketone bodies in the blood of pregnant women in the last trimester of pregnancy only 12–18 hours after fasting.

It has been noted that this accelerated production of ketone bodies may have a pathological effect on the course of labour and it has certainly been part of the routine observation of a labouring woman to test her urine for ketones. Work by Foulkes and Dumoulin (1983) and Sabata and co-workers (1968) suggests an association between the occurrence of ketosis and prolonged labour. A review of the evidence by Tricia Anderson (1998) explains ketosis as a physiological condition; it is evidence that the body is working effectively to provide energy for itself: ' the majority of sources seem to agree that ketosis is a physiological part of normal labour; therefore in the absence of other pathological findings it does not require treatment. It becomes pathological only by association when maternal or fetal acid-base status is compromised. It follows that we should not test for it routinely in labour; rather focus our efforts in looking for signs of maternal or fetal acidosis' (1998: 25).

Anderson also notes that as childbirth has moved from the home to the hospital environment, a new phenomenon, iatrogenic ketosis, may have occurred. Labouring women may become more markedly ketotic because they are not allowed to eat and drink as they wish. However, she also notes that 'force feeding' women could be equally detrimental, because of the evidence to suggest that elevated ketone and free fatty acid plasma levels are actually beneficial to the progress of labour.

What is the energy requirement of a woman in active labour?

The energy cost of active labour is said to be between 2.9 and 4.2 MJ (700–1000 cal) per hour, a tenfold increase over the average hourly expenditure during the third trimester (Ludka and Roberts, 1993). This is an often quoted figure which is disputed by some authors.

Hazle (1986) and Lewis (1991) referred to the labouring woman as a marathon runner. This would imply that the muscular activity of labour is great and that in order to fuel this activity, adequate oral intake is essential. Other writers (Odent, 1994; Anderson, 1998; and see Chapter 4 by McNabb in this volume) have suggested that the uterus, being a smooth muscle, works much more efficiently than skeletal muscle and does not make huge energy demands at all. It can utilize fatty acids and ketones readily as an energy source. It is also suggested that because the woman in physiological labour becomes withdrawn from higher cerebral activity and her skeletal muscles are at rest, her energy requirements are less than normal.

What is the fluid requirement for a labouring woman?

Poor fluid intake or increased losses from excessive sweating may result in dehydration. The normal healthy woman whose pregnancy is full term has an abundance of water, at least 2 litres in her expanded extracellular space. Whilst this may be thought sufficient to meet her needs during labour (Dumoulin and Foulkes, 1984), careful monitoring of fluid intake and output will prevent dehydration and the need for intravenous therapy.

One of the first symptoms of dehydration is fatigue. Greenleaf and co-workers (1983) showed that a 5% water loss can reduce normal physical work capacity by 20–30%. The mother's capacity to perform the arduous physical activity required during labour might be reduced if she is poorly hydrated. According to Dumoulin and Foulkes (1984), severe maternal ketosis together with starvation and fatigue can lead to inefficient uterine action. This may result in labour being artificially accelerated with intravenous drugs and fluids and may also increase the likelihood of instrumental delivery (Broach and Newton, 1988).

One of the recommendations made by Mendelson (1946) was 'withholding oral feeding during labour and substituting parenteral administration where necessary'. Obstetricians and midwives have observed the urine of labouring women for the presence of ketones and used this as an indicator of the need for intravenous fluid replacement. The wisdom of trying to replace food and fluid with intravenous solutions is certainly questionable.

There are a number of controlled research trials which are relevant, and are reviewed by Johnson and co-workers (1989). These reveal that there are several major disadvantages to the use of intravenous glucose solutions for rehydration, and prevention or treatment of ketonuria. The rise in maternal serum glucose (Inman, 1971; Ames *et al.*, 1975; Lawrence *et al.*,

1982; Morton *et al.*, 1985; Evans *et al.*, 1986) is accompanied by a rise in serum insulin (Morton *et al.*, 1985), and there is a corresponding effect in the fetus (Evans *et al.*, 1986; Inman, 1971; Lawrence *et al.*, 1982). The umbilical arterial blood pH may also be decreased (Inman, 1971; Lawrence, 1982). The fetus can suffer from hyperinsulinaemia, resulting in neonatal hypoglycaemia. The excessive use of salt-free intravenous infusions can result in hyponatraemia in both mother and fetus (Tarnow-Mordi *et al.*, 1981).

In this chapter, we have addressed some of the principles that any health professional or pregnant woman might apply when considering the issues around eating and drinking in labour. There has been very little research looking at the effects of particular food and fluid intake on labour progress and outcome, and there is no published work to confirm the nutritional needs of a labouring woman (Johnson, 1989).

There also appear to be opposing views about the physiological energy use of a woman in labour. On the one hand she could be likened to an athlete running a marathon, with her uterine muscle contracting strongly and rhythmically, and her mind concentrating hard on coping with the pain and her breathing deep. An athlete who has poor energy and fluid intake will give a poor performance; cannot the same be said for the fasted labouring woman?

On the other hand, the uterine muscle is an involuntary organ composed of striated muscle which both stores and uses its energy supply very efficiently. It is also able to make use of ketone bodies for fuel and may not consume the vast amounts of energy we assume in the above picture.

If we choose to look at each woman as an individual, some will be more physically active than others in labour, just as some women want to eat and drink and others do not. We need to apply the knowledge we have about the digestive system and the effects of different foodstuffs on it, in order to offer those women who choose to eat and drink, the appropriate things.

Using the points raised in the previous discussion, foods and drinks which fit the following criteria would be suitable for labouring women:

- help to maintain a high LOS pressure
- are smooth in consistency
- will leave the stomach rapidly
- will not increase gastric acidity.

The policy discussed by Newton and Champion (1997) graded parturiants as high or low risk. Women who were considered high risk were allowed clear fluids only whilst those regarded as low risk were able to eat and drink from a restricted range of food with the following characteristics:

- low fat
- high carbohydrate/high energy content
- low residue (fibre)
- homogeneous, liquid or semi-liquid
- near iso-osmolar
- neutral pH
- neutral temperature
- cheap, convenient and tasty.

Suggestions for foods and drinks which fulfil these criteria are listed in Tables 3.2 and 3.3.

Table 3.2 Drinks for women in labour

Low fat yoghurt drinks
Fresh fruit juices (long life drinks, especially apple, lemon, pineapple, tend to be more acidic)
Tea with skimmed milk
Soups (tomato, chicken, beef)
Squash drinks (not too concentrated)
Water
Naturally carbonated mineral waters

Source: Newton and Champion, 1997

Table 3.3 Foods for women in labour

Low fat, low residue, and well chewed: e.g.
Toast with low fat spread, jam, honey
Cereals with skimmed milk
Plain biscuits
Small can of smooth soup
Chocolate wafer biscuit
Low fat, lump free yoghurt or fromage frais

Source: Newton and Champion, 1997

To conclude, the most recent work about oral intake in labour by Scrutton *et al.* (1999: 333) suggests that '*isotonic drinks* which have been shown to be rapidly emptied from the stomach and absorbed by the gastro-intestinal tract may provide an alternative nutritional strategy in labour'.

References

Ames, A.C., Cobbold, S. and Maddock, J. (1975) Lactic acidosis complicating treatment of ketosis of labour. *British Medical Journal* 4: 611–13

Anderson, T. (1998) Is ketosis in labour pathological? *The Practising Midwife* 1 (9): 22–6

Atkinson, R., Rushman, G.B. and Alfred Lee, J (eds) (1987) *A Synopsis of Anaesthesia*. London: Bailliere Tindall

Bainbridge, E.T., Temple, J.G., Nicholas, S.P., Newton, J.R. and Boriah, V. (1983) Symptomatic gastro-oesophageal reflux in pregnancy. A comparative study of white Europeans and Asians in Birmingham. *British Journal of Clinical Practice* 37: 53–7

Broach, J. and Newton, N. (1988) Food and beverages in labor. Part 1: Cross-cultural and historical practices. *Birth* 15 (2): 81–5

Carp, H., Jayaram, A. and Stoll, M. (1992) Ultrasound examination of the stomach contents of parturiants. *Anaesthesia and Analgesia* 74: 683–7

COMA (A) (1991) *Department of Health Report on Health and Social Subjects 41: Dietary Reference Values for Food Energy and Nutrients in the UK.* London: HMSO, p. 2.4.1

COMA (B) (1991) *Department of Health Report on Health and Social Subjects 41:Dietary Reference Values for Food Energy and Nutrients in the UK.* London: HMSO, p. xix

Davenport, H. (1982) *Physiology of the Digestive Tract.* Chicago: Yearbook Medical Publications

Dumoulin, J. and Foulkes, J. (1984) Ketonuria during labour (commentary). *British Journal of Obstetrics and Gynaecology*, 91: 97–8

Escott-Stump, S. (1992) *Nutrition in Diagnosis Related Care,* 3rd edition. Philadelphia: Febiger, p. 27

Evans, S.E., Crawford, J.S., Stevens, I.D., Durbin, G.M. and Daya, H. (1986) Fluid therapy for induced labour under epidural analgesia: biochemical consequences for mother and infant. *British Journal of Obstetrics and Gynaecology* 93: 329–33

Felig, P., Kim, Y., Lynch, V. and Hendler, R. (1972) Amino acid metabolism during starvation and pregnancy. *Journal of Clinical Investigation* 51: 1195–202

Foulkes, J. and Dumoulin, J. (1983) Ketosis in labour. *British Journal of Hospital Medicine* 29 (6): 562–4

Greenleaf, J.E., Brock, P.S., Keil, L.C. and Morse, J.T. (1983) Drinking and water balance during exercise and heat acclimation. *Journal of Applied Physiology: Respiratory, Environmental and Exercise Physiology* 54: 414–19

Hazle, N.R. (1986) Hydration in labour: is routine intravenous hydration necessary? *Journal of Nurse Midwifery* 31: 171

Hester, J.B. and Heath, M.L. (1977) Pulmonary acid aspiration syndrome: should prophylaxis be routine? *British Journal of Anaesthesia* 49: 595–9

Hill, G.L. (1992) *Disorders of Nutrition and Metabolism in Clinical Surgery*, Part 1. London: Churchill Livingstone, pp. 7–8

Holdsworth, J.D. (1978) The place of amorphine prior to obstetric analgesia. *Journal of International Medical Research* 6: 26–32

Howard, F.A. and Sharp, D.S. (1973) Effect of metoclopramide on gastric emptying during labour. *British Medical Journal* 1: 446–8

Inman, S.E. (1971) The treatment of ketosis in labour. *Journal of Obstetrics and Gynaecology of the British Commonwealth* 78: 624–7

Johnson, C., Keirse, M.J.N.C., Enkin, M. and Chalmers, I. (1989) Nutrition and hydration in labour. In I. Chalmers, M. Enkin and M.J.N.C. Keirse (eds) *Effective Care in Pregnancy and Childbirth*. Oxford: Oxford University Press, pp. 827–32

Lawrence, G.F., Brown, V.A., Parsons, R.J. and Cooke, I.D. (1982) Feto-maternal consequences of high dose glucose infusion during labour. *British Journal of Obstetrics and Gynaecology* 89: 27–32

Lewis, P. (1991) Food for thought – should women fast or feed in labour? *Modern Midwife* July / August: 14–17

Ludka, L.M. (1987) *Fasting During Labor. International Confederation of Midwives 21st Congress Proceedings*, The Hague, August 1987. *Katilolehti* 93 (6): 25–8

Ludka, L.M. and Roberts, C.C. (1993) Eating and drinking in labor: a literature review. *Journal of Nurse-Midwifery* 38 (4): 199–207

Mendelson, C.L. (1946) The aspiration of stomach contents into the lungs during obstetric anaesthesia. *American Journal of Obstetrics and Gynecology* 52: 191–205

Moir, D. and Thornburn, J. (1986) *Obstetric Anaesthesia and Analgesia*. London: Bailliere Tindall

Morton, K.E., Jackson, M.C. and Gillmer, M.D.G. (1985) A comparison of the effects of four intravenous solutions for the treatment of ketonuria during labour. *British Journal of Obstetrics and Gynaecology* 92: 473–9

Murphy, D.F., Nally, B., Gardener, J. and Unwin, A. (1984) Effect of metoclopramide on gastric emptying before elective and emergency caesarean section. *British Journal of Anaesthesia* 56: 1113–16

Newton, C. and Champion, P. (1997) Oral intake in labour: Nottingham's policy formulated and audited. *British Journal of Midwifery* 5 (7): 418–22

Nimmo, W.S., Wilson, J. and Prescott, L.F. (1975) Narcotic analgesics and delayed gastric emptying in labour. *The Lancet* i: 890–3

Odent, M. (1994) Laboring women are not marathon runners. *Midwifery Today* 31: 23–51

O'Reilly, S., Hoyer, P. and Walsh, E. (1993) Low risk mothers: oral intake and emesis in labour. *Journal of Nursing Midwifery* 38(4): 228–35

Richardson, C.T., Walsh, J.H. and Hicks, M.I. (1976) Studies on the mechanism of food stimulated gastric acid secretion in normal human subjects. *Journal of Clinical Investigation* 58: 623–31

Roberts, R.B. and Shirley, M.A. (1976) The obstetrician's role in reducing the risk of aspiration pneumonitis with particular reference to the use of oral antacids. *American Journal of Obstetrics and Gynaecology* 124: 611–17

Rombeau, J.L. and Cauldwell, M.D. (1984) *Enteral and Tube Feeding*. Philadelphia: W.B. Saunders, pp. 23–4

Sabata, V., Wolf, H. and Lausmann, S. (1968) The role of free fatty acids, glycerol, ketone bodies and glucose in the energy metabolism of the mother and fetus during delivery. *Biologia Neonatorum* 13 (1): 7–17

Scrutton, M.J.L., Metcalfe, G.A., Lowry, C., Seed, P.T. and O'Sullivan, G. (1999) Eating in labour. *Anaesthesia* 54: 329–34

Smith, I.D. and Bogod, D.G. (1995) Feeding in labour. *Bailliere's Clinical Anaesthesiology* 9 (4): 735–47

Tarnow-Mordi, W.O., Shaw, J.C.L., Liu, D., Gardner, D.A. and Flynn F.V. (1981) Iatrogenic hyponatraemia of the newborn due to maternal fluid overload: a prospective study. *British Medical Journal* 283: 639–42

Wilson, J. (1978) Gastric emptying in labour: Some recent findings and their clinical significance. *Journal of International Medical Research* 6 (Supplement 1): 54–60

Changes in maternal food appetite and metabolism in labour and the shift from fetal to neonatal metabolism

Mary McNabb

- Pregnancy has a profound effect upon maternal food appetite and metabolism which provides a fairly constant level of nutrients for the fetus across the fed–fasted cycle
- The placenta is completely permeable to ketone bodies, which provide the fetus with growth and energy requirements during maternal fasting. The fetus is able to utilize ketone bodies efficiently in a variety of tissues including the brain
- Oxytocin is a key regulator of appetite, thirst and ingestive behaviours. Oxytocin stimulates prolactin secretion in late pregnancy and early labour and also decreases maternal appetite and gastrointestinal activity via central and peripheral mechanisms during active labour
- Elevated levels of prolactin in the early part of labour may stimulate maternal appetite. Around 2 hours prior to birth prolactin levels fall dramatically and the pulsatile release of oxytocin becomes more frequent and seems to induce a fall in maternal appetite during active labour
- Hormonal changes in labour also stimulate a fall in

maternal and fetal glucose levels

- Evidence suggests that the ability of the baby to metabolize lipids following birth is stimulated by transplacental supplies of ketones and inhibited by elevated concentrations of glucose
- Emotional stress during labour seems to raise maternal glucose levels which has negative implications for the transition from carbohydrate to lipid metabolism that occurs in the neonate immediately after birth

Introduction

From the 1970s, clinical studies began to reveal maternal, fetal and neonatal morbidity associated with the twin policy of food withdrawal and intravenous electrolyte solutions that was introduced as an essential component of active management of labour. Research findings emerged on the risks of intravenous fluid overload given the plasma volume expansion and reduced diuresis that characterizes labour (Tarnow-Mordi *et al.*, 1981; Mendiola *et al.*, 1982; Lind, 1983; Singhi and Chookango, 1984). Findings on pharmacological antacids also led to questions about the efficacy of many preparations, as neutralizing buffers, while other studies showed a positive association between prolonged fasting and increased gastric fluid volume, with a lower pH (Miller *et al.*, 1983; Roberts and Shirley, 1976, 1980).

By the 1980s and 1990s, general anaesthesia was no longer used for pain control during birth and general anaesthesia for caesarean sections also began to decline. At the same time safer induction techniques became standard practice, making anaesthesia a rare cause of either maternal mortality or morbidity (Parker, 1954; Crawford, 1956; Elkington, 1991). Taken together, these events have encouraged midwives, obstetricians and anaesthetists to re-examine the potential risks of prolonged fasting and consider the introduction of safe oral intake policies in labour (Crawford, 1956; Elkington, 1991; Smith and Bogod, 1995; Tourangeau *et al.*, 1999).

To contribute to an independent perspective on maternal food appetite and gastrointestinal functions during labour, this chapter will examine adaptations in food ingestion, gastrointestinal and metabolic functions in relation to nutritional and hormonal regulation of fetal growth, and the transition from carbohydrate to lipid metabolism immediately following birth (Uvnas-Moberg, 1989; Prip-Buus *et al.*, 1995; Pegorier *et al.*, 1998; Herrera and Amudquivar, 2000).

Neurohormonal regulation of ingestion and metabolism

In the non-pregnant state appetite and energy homeostasis are tightly regulated by oroxigenic and anoroxigenic signals that connect key hormonal secretions in peripheral organs with brain stem and hypothalamic neurones. Central and peripheral oroxigenic signals include neuropeptide Y (NPY), β-endorphin, noradrenaline, galanin, prolactin, growth hormone (GH) and ghrelin, a recently discovered brain-gut peptide that is released from the stomach in response to fasting (Kojima *et al.*, 1999; Tschop *et al.*, 2000; Nakazato *et al.*, 2001). Within the hypothalamus, NPY seems to be an essential component integrating energy homeostasis across the circadian cycle. This neuropeptide is a potent appetite stimulator and has synergistic and regulatory interactions with a number of other oroxigenic signals including ghrelin, β-endorphin, galanin and γ-aminobutyric acid (GABA) (Kalra *et al.*, 1999; Tschop *et al.*, 2000). When injected centrally ghrelin has a potent effect on appetite while peripheral daily administration stimulates GH secretion and adiposity in rodents (Kalra *et al.*, 1999; Morien *et al.*, 1999; Kojima *et al.*, 1999; Tschop *et al.*, 2000; Nakazato *et al.*, 2001). In a variety of experimental models, prolactin (PRL) and GH stimulate food intake, fat deposition, weight gain, islet beta-cell proliferation and insulin secretion (Gustafson *et al.*, 1980; Quigley *et al.*, 1982; Gerardo-Gettens *et al.*, 1989; Byatt *et al.*, 1993; Noel and Woodside, 1993; Brelje *et al.*, 1994; Heil, 1999; Freemark *et al.*, 2001).

Under basal conditions, glucocorticoids interact with NPY and noradrenaline to promote ingestion and metabolism of carbohydrates and fats across the circadian cycle (Tempel and Leibowitz, 1994). In contrast, stress induced activation of hypothalamic–pituitary–adrenocortical (HPA) axis hormones inhibit food intake, gastric motility and gastric acid secretion and stimulate colonic propulsion (Coskun *et al.*, 1997; Kern *et al.*, 1997; Heinrichs and Richards, 1999; Martinez and Tache, 2001). Outside of the anorexigenic effects of stress-induced corticotrophin-releasing hormone (CRH), leptin, α-melanocyte-stimulating hormone (α-MSH), serotonin, dopamine, oestrogen, cholecystokinin (CCK) and oxytocin inhibit food intake and induce satiety (Lieverse *et al.*, 1995; Flanagan-Cato *et al.*, 1998; Ahima *et al.*, 2000; Diaz-Cabiale *et al.*, 2000; Wauters *et al.*, 2000; Wirth *et al.*, 2001; Hay-Schmidt *et al.*, 2001). Of these, leptin has emerged as a key regulator of body weight and adipose tissue. This peptide hormone is produced in adipocytes and studies indicate a strong positive correlation between serum leptin concentrations and the amount of body fat.

Within the hypothalamus, leptin inhibits food intake and regulates energy expenditure and thermogenesis, to maintain a constant amount of stored body fat (Wauters *et al.*, 2000). In appetite regulation, leptin inhibits NPY, α-MSH and a variety of glucose-sensitive neurones and amplifies the satiating potency of CCK (Emond *et al.*, 2001; Kokkotou *et al.*, 2001). During pregnancy, leptin concentrations increase in association with the rise in adipose tissue. However, this is not associated with decreased food intake or a decline in metabolic efficiency and current findings suggest that pregnancy and lactation induce a state of leptin resistance (Holness *et al.*, 1999; Rump *et al.*, 2001).

Oxytocin, ingestion and metabolism

Experiments on dogs, pigs, calves and dairy cows have demonstrated that a pulsatile pattern of oxytocin release coincides with ingestive behaviours and episodes of suckling and milking (Uvnas-Moberg *et al.*, 1985; Verbalis *et al.*, 1986; Lindstrom *et al.*, 2001). In all animals, feeding- and suckling-induced oxytocin release is characterized by brief pulses that often commence just before ingestion begins. In calves and dairy cows, oxytocin concentration seems to be positively associated with the duration of feeding behaviours (Lindstrom *et al.*, 2001). This finding indicates that sensory nerves in the oral mucosa that are stimulated during suckling, chewing and swallowing, along with feeding related release of gastrointestinal hormones may mediate oxytocin release in the paraventricular nucleus, by vagal sensory pathways activated by the presence of food in the gut (Verbalis *et al.*, 1991). Through this mechanism, gastrointestinal hormones like cholecystokinin (CCK) may stimulate oxytocin inducing satiety and sedation following meals (Verbalis *et al.*, 1986; Uvnas-Moberg, 1994).

Experiments on rats have found that central administration of microgram doses of oxytocin have an inhibitory effect on food and salt ingestion and gastric motility but when central administration of microgram doses or subcutaneous administration of milligram doses is repeated over 3–5 days, oxytocin has a stimulatory effect on weight gain, in selected strains, that seems to be mediated by higher levels of CCK and insulin (Olson *et al.*, 1991a, 1991b; Flanagan *et al.*, 1992; Verbalis *et al.*, 1993, 1995; Bjorkstrand and Uvnas-Moberg, 1996; Uvnas-Moberg *et al.*, 1996, 1998; Lokrantz *et al.*, 1997). Other experiments on rats have found that peripheral oxytocin has a direct stimulatory effect on glucagon secretion, adipose tissue metabolism and fluid homeostasis, including renal handling of salt and water, in conjunction with vasopressin and atrial natriuretic peptide (ANP) (Hanif *et al.*, 1982; Krahn *et al.*, 1986; Siaud *et al.*, 1991; Widmaier *et al.*, 1991; Blackburn *et al.*, 1992; Byatt *et al.*, 1993; Bull *et al.*, 1994; Haanwinckel *et al.*, 1995; Bjorkstrand *et al.*, 1996; Windle *et al.*, 1997). Taken together, these findings indicate that food appetite, thirst, ingestive behaviours, fluid homeostasis and metabolism are regulated by diverse patterns of oxytocin release that are activated in different physiological states (Verbalis *et al.*, 1986; Olson *et al.*, 1991c; Uvnas-Moberg, 1997; Leng *et al.*, 1999; Verbalis, 1999; Diaz-Cabiale *et al.*, 2000; Gimpl and Fahrenholz, 2001).

Oxytocin – glucose homeostasis and insulin secretion

Evidence from human and animal studies suggests that oxytocin has some role in the regulation of glucose homeostasis (Fisher *et al.*, 1987; Widmaier, 1991; Chiodera *et al.*, 1992; Altszuler and Fuchs, 1994; Bjorkstrand *et al.*, 1996; Briski and Brandt, 2000). In adults, glucoprivation stimulates central oxytocin release while *in vitro* evidence suggests that hyperglycaemia inhibits oxytocin secretion (Fisher *et al.*, 1987; Widmaier *et al.*, 1991; Chiodera *et al.*, 1992; Briski and Brandt, 2000). In the fasted state, peripheral injections of oxytocin stimulate a significant rise in plasma glucose and glucagon and a transient increase in insulin (Altszuler and Hampshire, 1981; Vilhardt *et al.*, 1986; Stock *et al.*, 1990). Short term food deprivation in lactating rats has also been shown to stimulate a significant rise in circulating oxytocin and episodes of suckling are followed by a significant increase in glucose and glucagon (Widmaier *et al.*, 1991; Bjorkstrand *et al.*, 1992; Bjorkstrand *et al.*, 1996).

In the fed state, oxytocin neurones from the paraventricular nucleus may have a dual effect on insulin secretion, through interactions with the dorsal motor nucleus of the vagus and the nucleus tractus solitarus in the medulla, while peripheral oxytocin has been shown to augment glucose induced insulin secretion (Knudtzon, 1983; Gao *et al.*, 1991; Siaud *et al.*, 1991; Bjorkstrand *et al.*, 1996). In the fed state, administration of nanogram doses of oxytocin into the lateral ventricle have a stimulatory effect on insulin that seems to be mediated by the vagus nerve (Bjorkstrand *et al.*, 1996) while nanogram doses into the dorsal motor nucleus of the vagus have an inhibitory effect that is reversed by an oxytocin antagonist (Siaud *et al.*, 1991). Taken together these findings suggest that central oxytocin neurones may regulate glucose homeostasis through dual pathways between the paraventricular nucleus and the medulla.

To understand the effects of maternal food appetite and glucose levels in active labour on the transition from fetal to neonatal metabolism, the influences of oxytocin on maternal food appetite, gastrointestinal function, glucose homeostasis and adipose tissue metabolism will be examined, in relation to the hormonal changes that occur during late pregnancy and labour.

Pregnancy – maternal appetite, digestion and metabolism

During early pregnancy, food appetite is characterized by recurrent episodes of intense hunger, nausea and vomiting which tends to persist in varying degrees throughout pregnancy and labour (Lacroix *et al.*, 2000). At the same time, characteristic changes occur in food preferences and these persist to some extent throughout pregnancy. Recent research on well-nourished women suggests that nausea, vomiting and reduced energy intake in early pregnancy are positively associated with preconceptual body mass index; increased placental size and infant birthweight while experimental studies on well-nourished sheep suggest that reduced energy intake in early pregnancy stimulates placental growth and birthweight (Slen, 1969; Tierson *et al.*, 1986; Godfrey *et al.*, 1996; Huxley, 2000).

Digestion and absorption are enhanced during pregnancy and lactation by decreased gastrointestinal motility; enlargement of the duodenal villi; prolonged transit time in the small intestine that increases as pregnancy advances, and enhanced absorption of glucose, lipids, amino acids, calcium, iron, sodium/chloride and water (Hytten, 1980; Lawson *et al.*, 1985; Barrett *et al.*, 1994; Kovacs and Kronenberg, 1997; Zhu *et al.*, 1998; Condliffe *et al.*, 2001). Many of these changes seem to be regulated by rising levels of insulin, PRL, GH, placental lactogen (PL), oestrogen, progesterone and by an increased parasympathetic tone, although data remain incomplete and contradictory findings have been reported on gastrointestinal peptides and gastric acid secretion (Hytten, 1980; Lawson *et al.*, 1985; Baird, 1986; Hornnes and Kuhl, 1986; Linden *et al.*, 1987; Uvnas-Moberg, 1989; Freemark *et al.*, 2001).

Increased glucose induced insulin secretion in early pregnancy stimulates maternal anabolism while progesterone, prolactin and GH act centrally to increase maternal appetite and changing concentrations of oestrogen and progesterone may operate with the adipose-brain hormone leptin to reset hypothalamic control of energy balance that stimulates an increase and subsequent decline in maternal adipose tissue stores with a characteristic distribution peculiar to pregnancy and lactation (Hervey, 1969; Rebuffe-Schrive *et al.*, 1985; Baird, 1986; Gerardo-Gettens *et al.*, 1989; Fraser, 1991; Byatt *et al.*, 1993; Sivan *et al.*, 1998; Stock and Bremme, 1998; Varma *et al.*, 1999). In the periphery, progesterone reduces gastrointestinal motility and may operate with CCK and somatostatin, to reduce gastric emptying time and also with PRL and PL to enhance glucose stimulated insulin secretion and fat deposition (Linden *et al.*, 1987; Sorenson *et al.*, 1987; Uvnas-Moberg, 1989; Freemark *et al.*, 2001).

Maternal, placental and fetal metabolism

For mother and fetus, the latter half of pregnancy marks a very distinct period of metabolic transition. Maternal weight gain slows down, while that of the fetus accelerates. Fetal growth velocity increases between 18 and 34 weeks' gestation and then continues at a considerably slower rate towards term (Moore and Persaud, 1993). From 26 to 40 weeks' gestation, fetal weight increases more than fourfold and by term, fat accumulation accounts for over 90% of calories consumed by the fetus (Feldman *et al.*, 1992). While overall fetal weight gain increases more slowly from around 34 weeks of gestation, the rate of fat accretion is approximately linear between

36 and 40 weeks and the brain also exhibits a linear growth pattern during the last trimester and continues growing at a slower rate, until 18–24 months (Dobbing and Sands, 1973; Innis, 1991; Van Aerde *et al.*, 1998).

From around 35 weeks of pregnancy, the earlier maternal tendency to accumulate adipose tissue diminishes and stores begin to decline as enhanced adipose tissue lipolysis becomes a characteristic feature of *both* fed and fasted states (Flint *et al.*, 1979; Herrera *et al.*, 1987; Dutta-Roy, 1997; Haggarty *et al.*, 1999; Sidebottom *et al.*, 2001). The altered pattern of fetal growth during the last trimester is accompanied by a rapid rise in transplacental supply of fatty acids and ketone bodies; increased deposition of glycogen in a number of organs, including hepatic, skeletal muscle and adipose tissue; increased accretion of long- and short-chain fatty acids, in adipose, hepatic and brain tissue and a decline in the weight-specific consumption of glucose (Jones, 1976; Herrera *et al.*, 1988; Uauy *et al.*, 1989; Schneider, 1996; Haggarty *et al.*, 1997; Haggarty *et al.*, 1999; Herrera, 2000).

Maternal metabolism – fed and fasted states

In the second half of pregnancy, longitudinal glucose tolerance tests on Western populations reveal a greater and more prolonged hyperglycaemia in the fed state compared to non-pregnant and early pregnant values. This metabolic shift is accompanied by a large increase in glucose stimulated insulin secretion (Fraser, 1991). In relation to lipid metabolism, the latter half of pregnancy is characterized by increased intestinal absorption of triacylglycerol (TG) and hepatic esterification of free fatty acids, along with diminished lipid accumulation and enhanced mobilization of adipose tissue stores (Flint *et al.*, 1979; Knopp *et al.*, 1981; Besnard *et al.*, 1995). *In vitro* studies on adipose tissue suggest a significant fall in fatty acid formation from circulating glucose and increased formation of fatty acids from TG stores, independent of the availability of glucose (Knopp *et al.*, 1970; Elliot, 1975).

During the fasted state, most findings indicate that plasma glucose concentrations decline progressively as pregnancy advances and there is an accelerated activation of lipolysis significantly above that observed in the fed state (Knopp *et al.*, 1970; Freinkel, 1980; Herrera *et al.*, 1990; Fraser, 1991; Mills *et al.*, 1998). Overall, less maternal glucose gets converted to fatty acids while additional lipids are made available by increased absorption, hepatic synthesis and adipose tissue lipolysis. In both fed and fasted states, the second half of pregnancy is characterized by a physiological hyperlipidaemia that reflects maternal fatty acid intake, before and during pregnancy (Herrera *et al.*, 1988; Dutta-Roy, 1997; Raygada *et al.*, 1998; Haggarty *et al.*, 1999; Hornstra, 2000).

The increased glucose and lipids that become available as a result of these changes are utilized through specific alterations in the metabolic capacities of the liver, placenta and mammary in *both* fed and fasted states. During the second half of pregnancy, the placenta displays a progressive increase in the uptake of glucose *and* fatty acids; while the mammary gland and liver demonstrate a complementary pattern of increased uptake of fatty acids during *both* fed *and* fasted states (Flint *et al.*, 1979; Lopez-Luna, 1994; Dutta-Roy, 1997; Haggarty *et al.*, 1999; Sivan *et al.*, 1999).

Placental and fetal metabolism of glucose

The increased placental and fetal requirements for glucose during the second half of pregnancy are met by a rise in overall placental transport capacity and an increase in transplacental glucose concentration gradient which is thought to be due to a greater fall in fetal plasma glucose concentration relative to maternal concentrations (Hay, 1995). Serial studies on human infants have found that the maternal–fetal concentration gradient increases from mid-gestation to term (Bozzetti *et al.*, 1988). This seems to result from increased glucose clearance, secondary to increased insulin secretion and insulin sensitivity, because of increased number of receptors, particularly in the rapidly growing mass of adipose and muscle tissues (Simmons *et al.*, 1978; Kaplan, 1981; Sterman *et al.*, 1983; Hill and Milner, 1985; Bozzetti *et al.*, 1988; Fowden, 1989; Chaffin *et al.*, 1995).

Placental lipid metabolism

During the latter half of pregnancy, the placenta demonstrates a growing capacity to remove triacylglycerols from the maternal circulation and selectively remove particular groups of essential fatty acids, through its unique population of fatty acid binding proteins (P-FABP) (Campbell *et al.*, 1996; Dutta-Roy, 1997; Haggarty *et al.*, 1999). Results from animal studies suggest that the former is due to the increased expression of lipoprotein lipase which hydrolyses the TG component of circulating lipoproteins, to provide free fatty acids and glycerol for placental uptake and regulated transfer to the fetus (Herrera *et al.*, 1988; Haggarty *et al.*, 1999). Research on placental delivery of essential fatty acids suggests that a number of hormonal mechanisms are involved in a complicated process that selectively provides docosahexaenoic acid (n-3) and arachidonic acid (n-6) for the distinct requirements of placental metabolism and central nervous system development of the fetus during the third trimester (Dutta-Roy, 1997; Clandinin, 1999).

Interrelations between the liver and mammary gland

During the last trimester the mammary gland and liver demonstrate a growing capacity to remove triacylglycerols from the maternal circulation. Experimental evidence from rats has demonstrated increased hepatic expression of fatty acid binding proteins in late pregnancy (P-FABP) and lipoprotein lipase activity has been found to increase rapidly in the mammary gland in the fed state during the last trimester and further increases have also been found just prior to parturition (Ramirez *et al.*, 1983; Lopez-Luna *et al.*, 1994; Besnard *et al.*, 1995; Campbell *et al.*, 1996; Dutta-Roy, 1997; Haggarty *et al.*, 1999). This means that the diminished lipid accumulation and enhanced mobilization of adipose tissue stores that occurs during the fed state is accompanied by enhanced lipid accumulation in the mammary gland. This redirects high circulating triacylglycerols away from adipose tissue and into the gland for milk synthesis, in preparation for lactation (Knopp *et al.*, 1981; Herrera *et al.*, 1988; Lopez-Luna *et al.*, 1994). Recent evidence suggests that lipoprotein lipase activity in the mammary gland is stimulated by heightened insulin secretion and rising maternal prolactin that particularly characterizes the latter part of pregnancy (Ramirez *et al.*, 1983; Bandyopadhyay *et al.*, 1995; Ramos and Herrera, 1996; Sivan *et al.*, 1999).

During the fasted state, most longitudinal studies in women show a gradual fall in plasma glucose with advancing gestation, reaching around 4 mmol/l during the last trimester (Mills *et al.*, 1998). The simultaneous decline in glucose and insulin during the fasted state is accompanied by maximal stimulation of adipose tissue lipolysis and a fall in lipid uptake by the mammary gland (Lopez-Luna *et al.*, 1994). The rapid increase in circulating levels of non-esterified fatty acids (NEFA) during the fasted state in late pregnancy is thought to stimulate a rise in lipoprotein lipase activity in the liver (Lopez-Luna *et al.*, 1994; Igal *et al.*, 1998). From being an exporter of a variety of lipoprotein fractions during the fed state, the liver becomes a temporary acceptor of triacylglycerols and these are used as substrates for free fatty acid and ketone body synthesis, which then become available in preference to glucose as metabolic fuel for a variety of maternal and fetal tissues (Herrera *et al.*, 1988; Lopez-Luna *et al.*, 1994; Sivan *et al.*, 1999).

Placental transport of ketones

The complete permeability of the placenta to ketone bodies provides the fetus with additional substrates, which may be used as energetic fuels and lipogenic substrates during maternal fasting (Seccombe *et al.*, 1977; Schambaugh, 1985; Bougneres *et al.*, 1986; Harding and Evans, 1991). Concentrations of ketone bodies in the maternal circulation increase during the third trimester and positive correlations have been found between maternal and fetal concentrations, with a concentration gradient from mother to fetus (Paterson *et al.*, 1967; Sabata *et al.*, 1968). While the fetus has a very low capacity for ketogenesis, a number of fetal tissues, notably the brain, heart, liver, kidneys and brown adipose tissue, have been shown to express the enzymes required to utilize ketone bodies and their activity increases during periods of maternal fasting *or* when the mother is fed a diet high in lipids (Dahlquist *et al.*, 1972; Girard, 1975; Herrera *et al.*, 1992; Ghebremeskel *et al.*, 1999). As a result of these changes in maternal metabolism in late pregnancy, the placenta receives and selectively transports increasing supplies of essential fatty acids and ketones and maintains a fairly constant supply of glucose for the fetus across the fed-fasted state (Sangild, 1999).

Fetal metabolism – glycogenesis and lipogenesis

From as early as 9 weeks' gestation, glycogen is deposited in fetal tissues and increases significantly in placental and fetal tissues during the third trimester (Shelley and Bassett, 1975; Kaneta *et al.*, 1991; Philipps, 1992). While the largest glycogen store is found in the liver, after 24 weeks' gestation, glycogen is also deposited in a number of tissues including, adipose and brain tissue, skeletal and cardiac muscle, lungs and intestines (Shelly, 1961; Sperling, 1994). By term, the well-nourished fetus has two to three times more glycogen in skeletal muscle and ten times more in cardiac muscle, compared to the adult (Page *et al.*, 1981).

Fat accretion in the human fetus is greater than in all other land based mammals, but in contrast to many other species, brown fat makes up only 3–6% of total adipose tissue (Battaglia, 1978). Between 26 and 30 weeks' gestation, non-fat and fat calories contribute equally to the energy content of the fetus. After 30 weeks, fat accumulation far exceeds the non-fat components and by term fat deposition accounts for more than 90% of calories accumulated (Heim, 1983; Tu and Tuch, 1997; Van Aerde *et al.*, 1998). The main lipogenic substrates are maternally derived glucose and fatty acids. The fetus displays an increasing capacity for lipid synthesis from glucose with advancing gestation and converts approximately 70% of glucose uptake to fat (Van Aerde *et al.*, 1998).

The increasing fetal capacity for glycogenesis and lipogenesis seems to largely be regulated by rising levels of insulin, PRL, PL and cortisol in the fetal circulation. As well as the increased expression of insulin receptors, prolactin receptors also increase in a variety of organs, including the liver, pancreas and adipose tissue, and these have been shown to function as a high affinity binding protein for PL, PRL and GH in a variety of organ systems (Symonds *et al.*, 1998; Freemark, 1999a, 1999b; Bispham *et al.*, 1999; Phillips *et al.*, 1999; Fleenor *et al.*, 2000; Phillips *et al.*, 2001). Insulin stimulates hepatic lipogenesis while insulin and cortisol induce the expression of enzymes required for glycogenesis (M'Zali *et al.*, 1997; Freemark, 1999a). PL and insulin stimulate placental glycogenesis and PRL and PL have been shown to have a direct lipogenic effect on adipose cells (Barash *et al.*, 1983; Freemark, 1999a).

Feto-placental regulation of maternal and fetal metabolism

The fetus is essentially a parenterally nourished organism receiving a fairly constant supply of simple nutrients from the maternal circulation across the feto-placental barrier. During this period of enhanced anabolic metabolism, the placenta selectively provides large amounts of glucose and amino acids and relatively small amounts of fatty acids from the maternal circulation (Girard *et al.*, 1992). While suckling and swallowing mechanisms are present during the third trimester, the intake of luminal nutrients remains very small compared to that transferred across the placenta (Roberts *et al.*, 2000). Consequently, minimal development occurs in exocrine pancreatic cells and there is no requirement for endocrine cells to regulate pre- and post-feeding cycles, as the feto-placental unit regulates maternal metabolism to supply a progressive increase in glucose, amino acids, essential and non-essential fatty acids across the fed–fasted cycle (Nolan and Proietto, 1994; Sangild, 1999).

Developmental changes in the fetal pancreas

Differentiation, proliferation, apoptosis and maturation occur in exocrine and endocrine cells during fetal and neonatal development (Sangild, 1999; Hill *et al.*, 2000; Kassem *et al.*, 2000; Sjoholm *et al.*, 2000). The initial formation of the pancreatic diverticulum is followed by cell differentiation. In the human fetus, this process commences at around 9 weeks' gestation, with rapid, interrelated differentiation of endocrine α-glucagon secreting cells and exocrine acini cells followed by the appearance of somatostatin releasing cells. A smaller number of β-cells have been observed by 10 weeks' gestation. At this stage of development, some β-cells are found alongside α-cells and most endocrine cells are either dispersed in the exocrine parenchyma or situated in small buds originating from the epithelium of minute ducts (Van Assche *et al.*, 1984; Sperling, 1994).

Endocrine cells predominate in the central portion of each lobe as only minimal acinar development takes place before the perinatal period (Singled, 1999). During the last 4–6 weeks of gestation, rapid growth occurs in the intestinal mucosa under the stimulatory influence of insulin and this is accompanied by acinar growth and increased synthesis of pancreatic enzymes, in preparation for the shift from parenteral to enteral feeding (Pang *et al.*, 1985; Menard *et al.*, 1999; Sangild, 1999). Before and during labour, fetal cortisol accelerates differentiation of gastric epithelial cells; stimulates gastrin and gastric acid secretion and regulates the processing of lipoproteins in the small intestine, facilitating digestion and uptake of milk lipids from the mammary gland following birth (Sangild *et al.*, 1995).

Development of pancreatic β-cells

In the human fetus, insulin is present in the pancreas from 8–9 weeks' gestation and increases eight- to tenfold between 17 and 32 weeks' gestation (Van Assche *et al.*, 1984; Fleenor *et al.*, 2000). β-cell proliferation is high from around 20 weeks and progressively declines from 32 weeks to reach very low levels at 6 months postpartum while apoptosis or cell death begins at very low levels at around 20 weeks, peaks around the time of birth and declines over the first two months postpartum (Tornehave and Larsson, 1997; Kassem *et al.*, 2000). By six months of age, both proliferation and apoptosis have reached very low levels and β-cell distribution approaches that in the adult (Kassem *et al.*, 2000). During this process of developmental apoptosis, glucose resistant fetal β-cells are gradually replaced by mature cells that begin to demonstrate a capacity for glucose dependent insulin secretion. In the human fetus this capacity does not appear before the third trimester (Sperling, 1994; Tu and Tuch, 1997; Fleenor *et al.*, 2000; Sjoholm *et al.*, 2000).

Current findings suggest that growth and proliferation of pancreatic β-cells is stimulated by glucose, amino acids, PL, PRL and GH. In a variety of studies during fetal and adult life glucose and amino acids have has been shown to stimulate β-cell growth and replication while *in vitro* experiments on mouse, rat and human fetal pancreatic tissue have found that GH, prolactin and PL induce β-cell growth and replication and promote the formation of islet-like cell clusters (Fleenor *et al.*, 2000; Sjoholm *et al.*, 2000). In cultured human pancreas at 12–21 weeks of gestation, PL and GH stimulate a 50% increase in insulin content and release in the presence of glucose (Freemark, 1999b).

Insulin and glucagon during fetal and early neonatal life

Insulin and glucagon have a number of unique developmental features in fetal and early neonatal life up to spontaneous weaning (Beard *et al.*, 1977; Sterman *et al.*, 1983;

Devaskar *et al.*, 1984; Hill and Milner, 1985; Bozzetti *et al.*, 1988; Lyonnet *et al.*, 1988; Fowden, 1989; Girard *et al.*, 1992; Macho *et al.*, 1995; Fowden *et al.*, 1999; Menard *et al.*, 1999). During the third trimester, circulating insulin levels rise and insulin concentrations in the fetus at term are much higher than in the adult (Ktorza *et al.*, 1985). In addition, the number and/or affinity of insulin receptors on a variety of tissues are higher than corresponding levels in the neonate and insulin receptors seem to be largely upregulated in response to hyperinsulinaemia while those in the neonate and adult are downregulated (Kaplan, 1981; Neufeld *et al.*, 1980). This means that the anabolic effects of insulin on fetal glucose, amino acid and fatty acid metabolism are enhanced by raised insulin secretion which in turn is regulated by basal maternal insulin and glucose concentrations (Bozzetti *et al.*, 1988; Langhoff-Roos *et al.*, 1989; Caruso *et al.*, 1998; Soltani, 1999).

During fetal and early neonatal life, glucagon does not seem to function as a physiological antagonist of insulin (Lawrence *et al.*, 1989). This is in marked contrast to the adult, where glucagon has a key role in regulating glucose metabolism, by stimulating glycogenolysis, gluconeogenesis and ketogenesis, in response to hypoglycaemia (Beaudry *et al.*, 1977; Devaskar *et al.*, 1984; Ktorza *et al.*, 1985). While glucagon is present in fetal plasma, at concentrations similar to maternal values, secretion is not noticeably modified by increases or decreases in circulating glucose (Chez *et al.*, 1974; Girard *et al.*, 1974; Lawrence *et al.*, 1989). Experimental studies on sheep have found that physiological doses of glucagon in late gestation produce no alteration or very modest increases in plasma glucose, while in the foal, pancreatic α-cells are functional but unresponsive to variations in plasma glucose in late gestation (Devaskar *et al.*, 1984; Lawrence *et al.*, 1989; Fowden *et al.*, 1999). In marked contrast to insulin, fetal glucagon receptors are fewer in number than in the adult and poorly connected to the membrane receptor. Taken together, these findings have led to the suggestion that the fetal liver has a physiological resistance to glucagon (Devaskar *et al.*, 1984; Lawrence *et al.*, 1989).

Hormonal regulation of nutrient metabolism – maternal compartment

Recent findings from a number of species suggest that PL, PRL and GH are selectively involved in regulating islet β-cell proliferation; insulin secretion; accumulation of adipose tissue stores, changes in glucose tolerance, lipolysis and growth and uptake of nutrient in the mammary gland, during pregnancy and lactation (Flint *et al.*, 1979; Brelje and Sorenson, 1991; Goodman *et al.*, 1991; Brelje *et al.*, 1993; Da Costa and Williamson, 1994; Brelje *et al.*, 1994; Bandyopadhyay *et al.*, 1995; Weinhaus *et al.*, 1998; Ramos *et al.*, 1999; Freemark *et al.*, 2001). Changing concentration of these hormones during pregnancy and labour seems to regulate maternal, fetal and neonatal adaptations in glucose and lipid metabolism in preparation for suckling and lactation.

In the maternal circulation, plasma levels of PL rise progressively from 3–4 weeks of gestation, reaching a peak of 5000–15 000 ng/ml several weeks before term, followed by a modest reduction before the onset of labour (Freemark, 1999b). Within the pituitary, a significant increase occurs in the number, size and secretory activity of prolactin-releasing cells accompanied by a simultaneous fall in the number and responsiveness of growth hormone-releasing cells (Yen, 1986; Frankenne *et al.*, 1988). From 10–25% of the total population in the non-pregnant state, lactotrophes grow to reach more than 50% during late pregnancy and lactation (Goluboff and Ezrin, 1969). Serum prolactin concentrations begin to rise during the luteal phase of the cycle and increase in a linear fashion to reach 10 times non-pregnant values at term (Yen, 1989, 1991; Nguyen *et al.*, 1997). Research evidence on primigravid and multigravid women suggests that these elevated levels are maintained during the first 6 hours of labour and then decline sharply, to reach their lowest values about 2 hours prior to birth (Rigg and Yen, 1977; Rigg *et al.*, 1977).

As happens in the non-pregnant state, an acute release of prolactin occurs in synchrony with food ingestion throughout pregnancy and prolactin is known to stimulate appetite in females in a dose-dependent manner (Quigley *et al.*, 1982; Gerardo-Gettens *et al.*, 1989; Yen, 1989; Sauve and Woodside, 1996; Heil, 1999). During the oestrus cycle, systemic and central infusion of prolactin stimulates increased food intake, fat deposition and weight gain (McGarry and Beck, 1962; Gerardo-Gettens *et al.*, 1989; Noel and Woodside, 1993; Freemark *et al.*, 2001). Chronic hyperprolactinaemia, as occurs in the second half of pregnancy, has been found to stimulate islet β-cell proliferation; decrease the glucose stimulation threshold for insulin secretion; modulate lipid metabolism in the liver and operate along with insulin to stimulate uptake of lipids by the mammary gland (Yen, 1989; Noel and Woodside, 1993; Ramos and Herrera, 1995; Weinhaus *et al.*, 1996; Igal *et al.*, 1998; Weinhaus *et al.*, 1998; Ramos *et al.*, 1999).

In contrast to prolactin, pituitary growth hormone (GH) is markedly suppressed during pregnancy. During the first trimester, GH is detectable in plasma but is unresponsive to many physiological stimuli and declines progressively as pregnancy advances (Eriksson *et al.*, 1989). From 15 weeks to term, it is gradually replaced by GH-V which becomes the major form of circulating GH in the maternal circulation (Frankenne *et al.*, 1988; Alsat *et al.*, 1997). GH-V differs from GH by 13 amino acid substitutions and has major sequence homology with PL and prolactin which have all evolved from a common precursor gene (Alsat *et al.*, 1997).

Because of these structural similarities, GH-V is thought to have similar influences on food intake, carbohydrate and lipid metabolism (Goodman and Coiro, 1981; Goodman and Grichting, 1983; Byatt *et al.*, 1993). *In vitro* evidence suggests that acute administration of GH and GH-V accelerates carbohydrate utilization while chronic administration decreases glucose uptake, stimulates insulin resistance and enhances lipolysis (Goodman *et al.*, 1991). Recent findings suggest that GH-V may play a key role in reorganizing maternal metabolism to sustain feto-placental growth and development during the latter half of pregnancy (Patel *et al.*, 1995; Zumkeller, 2000). In contrast to PL and prolactin, release of GH-V is stimulated by hypoglycaemia, suggesting that reduced availability of maternal glucose during the fasted state in the second half of pregnancy may inhibit maternal uptake of glucose and enhance adipose tissue lipolysis, to preserve nutrient availability for the fetus (Nolan and Proietto, 1994; Patel *et al.*, 1995).

Adaptations in the maternal endocrine pancreas

Current evidence suggests that the progressive rise in prolactin, placental growth hormone (GH-V) and PL directly stimulates a gradual increase in the number and responsiveness of maternal pancreatic islet β-cell population, until the end of pregnancy when the process is reversed by the combined effects of high concentrations of progesterone, oestrogen and glucocorticoids (Turtle and Kipnis, 1967; Fielder and Talamantes, 1987; Frankenne *et al.*, 1990; Philippe and Missotten, 1990; Lambillotte *et al.*, 1997; Chen *et al.*, 1998). *In vitro* evidence suggests that placental steroids, particularly progesterone, inhibit islet β-cell proliferation while glucocorticoids also stimulate apoptosis or cell death (Brelje *et al.*, 1993; Sorenson *et al.*, 1993; Weinhaus *et al.*, 1996; Weinhaus *et al.*, 2000).

These changes allow a progressive rise in glucose stimulated insulin secretion followed by a sharp decline during late pregnancy and labour. Following the period of enhanced maternal anabolism and insulin sensitivity in the first half of pregnancy, chronically elevated levels of GH-V, oestrogen and glucocorticoids, during the second half of pregnancy, seem to induce mild glucose intolerance, increased insulin resistance and rising plasma concentrations of free fatty acids (McGarry and Beck, 1962; Shamoon and Felig, 1974; Rigg and

Yen, 1977; Yen, 1989; Goodman *et al.*, 1991; Sivan *et al.*, 1999). *In vitro* evidence suggests that the insulin stimulating actions of PRL and PL and the lipolytic actions of GH-V and glucocorticoids are counteracted during the latter part of pregnancy by the more rapid rise in progesterone (Williams and Coultard, 1978; Sorenson *et al.*, 1993).

In human studies, circulating triacylglycerol concentrations decline between 40 weeks' gestation and two weeks postpartum and the degree of decline is most pronounced in women who are lactating (Darmady and Postle, 1982; Bandyopadhyay, 1995). Experimental studies on animals suggest that during late pregnancy and labour insulin secretion falls and circulating triglycerides begin to decline (Schams and Espanier, 1991; Martin-Hidalgo *et al.*, 1994). In rats, high maternal TG concentrations begin to decline during late pregnancy and labour, in association with a progressive rise in lipoprotein lipase activity in the mammary gland which is thought to be induced by high levels of insulin and prolactin (Flint *et al.*, 1979; Ramirez *et al.*, 1983; Martin-Hidalgo *et al.*, 1994; Ramos *et al.*, 1999). In a recent study on cows, peripheral concentrations of insulin declined during the last two days of pregnancy while concentrations in the mammary gland continued to rise until two days postpartum (Schams and Espanier, 1991). Taken together, these findings suggest that towards the end of pregnancy, hormonal stimulation of insulin secretion and hyperlipidaemia is modulated by the lipogenic actions of rising levels of progesterone and by the increased uptake of lipids by the mammary gland in preparation for lactation.

Changes in the maternal oxytocin system – pregnancy and labour

Considerable evidence on rats suggests that from mid pregnancy onwards, oxytocin neurones undergo extensive remodelling under the stimulatory influence of placental steroids. Towards the end of pregnancy, increased oxytocin mRNA and peptide have been demonstrated in a variety of brain nuclei both in and outside the hypothalamus while the content of oxytocin in the posterior pituitary gland increases by around 50% and a parallel rise occurs in central and peripheral receptor concentrations as pregnancy advances (Jirkowski *et al.*, 1989; Crowley *et al.*, 1995; Leng and Brown, 1997). Towards the end of pregnancy, oxytocin released from the median eminence into the anterior pituitary may indirectly increase maternal appetite, through its stimulatory action on prolactin (Noel and Woodside, 1993). The direct stimulatory effect of oxytocin on PRL secretion seems to operate during the last week of pregnancy and the first five hours of labour, when food appetite seems to increase (Crawford, 1956). Recent studies on rats suggest that oxytocin receptors on PRL-releasing cells increase dramatically at the end of pregnancy, allowing oxytocin to exert its full potential as a prolactin releasing factor before *and* after birth, as the stimulus for prolactin secretion switches from placenta to neonate (Kubota *et al.*, 1988; Brenton *et al.*, 1995).

Prolactin, GH-V and oxytocin – changes in maternal glucose and lipid metabolism in labour

In early labour GH-V levels decline followed by an equally sharp fall in prolactin around 2 hours prior to birth (Rigg and Yen, 1977; Mirlesse *et al.*, 1993). Taken together, these changes can be expected to dramatically enhance glucose tolerance and reduce insulin secretion, as labour progresses. At the same time, continuing high levels of placental oestrogen, progesterone and adrenal cortisol can be expected to maintain their combined inhibition of islet β-cell proliferation and insulin secretion (Golde *et al.*, 1982; Jovanovic and Peterson, 1983; Chen *et al.*, 1998; Weinhaus *et al.*, 2000).

Current *in vitro* evidence suggests that during periods when central oxytocin is stimulated, neurohypophyseal secretion into the peripheral circulation in the fasted state increases glucose production directly, by increasing hepatic glycogenolysis and gluconeogenesis while central and peripheral oxytocin increases glucose production by stimulating secretion of glucagon (Saudi *et al.*, 1991; Widmaier *et al.*, 1991; Altszuler *et al.*, 1992; Bjorkstrand *et al.*, 1996). In studies on rats, this glucoregulatory mechanism has been clearly demonstrated in adult male rats and in females during lactation (Widmaier *et al.*, 1991; Briski and Brandt, 2000). In males, the hypothalamic magnocellular neurones are transcriptionally activated in response to glucose substrate imbalance (Briski and Brandt, 2000). Male rats also display a significant increase in plasma glucose and glucagon following peripheral administration of 10 μg/kg oxytocin but in this experimental model no effect was observed following administration of oxytocin at 1 μg/kg (Widmaier *et al.*, 1991). At 12 days' lactation, significant correlations have been found between plasma glucose concentrations and endogenous oxytocin and peripheral concentrations of oxytocin rise significantly following a 24 hour fast, suggesting that oxytocin plays a key role in glucose homeostasis during lactation (Widmaier *et al.*, 1991; Bjorkstrand *et al.*, 1992, 1996).

In vitro studies also indicate that oxytocin has a dual mechanism of action in regulating adipose tissue metabolism (Muchmore *et al.*, 1981). In experiments on isolated rat adipocytes, doses of oxytocin below 10^{-8} mmol/l stimulate glucose oxidation, lipogenesis and glycogen synthesis and inhibit catecholamine stimulated lipolysis acting via the same receptor that is present in smooth muscle of the uterus and mammary gland (Hanif *et al.*, 1982; Mukherjee and Mukherjee, 1982). In contrast, at concentrations greater than 10^{-8} mmol/l oxytocin activates glucose transport while simultaneously inhibiting glycogen deposition and stimulating lipolysis (Muchmore *et al.*, 1981).

Current findings suggest that neurohypophyseal secretion of oxytocin in response to decreased systemic glucose availability persists during late pregnancy and labour (Douglas *et al.*, 1998; Briski and Brandt, 2000). In addition, the low plasma oxytocin concentrations of labour can be expected to improve glucose tolerance through the insulin-like effects on adipose tissue (Muchmore *et al.*, 1981; Fuchs *et al.*, 1991; Douglas *et al.*, 1998). During this period, oxytocin may largely supplant insulin as the combined inhibitory effects of placental steroids and glucocorticoids on insulin secretion are likely to be maintained during labour (Brelje *et al.*, 1993; Sorenson *et al.*, 1993; Weinhaus *et al.*, 1996, 2000). Both these mechanisms are compatible with clinical findings of a decline in fasting insulin levels between late pregnancy and birth and a sharp decline in insulin required by well-controlled diabetic women undergoing induction of labour with synthetic oxytocin (Golde *et al.*, 1982; Jovanovic and Peterson, 1983; Chen *et al.*, 1998). In the first of these studies, 48% of women did not need insulin in labour despite large requirements during pregnancy (Golde *et al.*, 1982). These findings strongly suggest that the insulin-like actions of low concentrations of oxytocin on adipose tissue along with the lipogenic effects of progesterone and the sharp decline in GH-V may explain the reduced insulin requirements observed in clinical studies on well-controlled diabetics (Golde *et al.*, 1982; Jovanovic and Peterson, 1983; Mirlesse *et al.*, 1993).

The progressive decline in circulating lipids from the end of pregnancy seems to be initiated by the more rapid rise in progesterone relative to GH-V and glucocorticoids and the increased uptake of fatty acids by the mammary gland in response to rising levels of insulin and prolactin (Flint *et al.*, 1979; Bandyopadhyay *et al.*, 1995; Ramos *et al.*, 1999). During labour, this trend is sustained by the sharp fall in GH-V coupled with the lipogenic actions of progesterone and the insulin-like actions of low concentrations of oxytocin on maternal adipose tissue (Rigg and Yen, 1977; Muchmore *et al.*, 1981; Hanif *et al.*, 1982; Mirlesse *et al.*, 1993; Martin-Hildago *et al.*, 1994). Taken together, these hormonal changes can be expected to induce a decline in basal maternal glucose levels during active labour with a correspondingly greater fall in glucose concentrations in the fetus (Bozzetti *et al.*, 1988).

Oxytocin, maternal food appetite and gastrointestinal function

In a number of experimental studies on fasted rats central administration of oxytocin inhibits food and salt ingestion in a dose-related manner (Krahn *et al.*, 1986; Arletti *et al.*, 1989; Olson *et al.*, 1991a; Siaud *et al.*, 1991; Blackburn *et al.*, 1992; Byatt *et al.*, 1993; Verbalis *et al.*, 1993, 1995; Bjorkstrand *et al.*, 1996; Coskun *et al.*, 1997; Windle *et al.*, 1997). In both fed and fasted states, similar treatment reversibly suppresses oral intake of glucose in a dose-related manner (Lokrantz *et al.*, 1997). Other experimental models have also demonstrated that central administration of oxytocin specifically decreases the stimulatory effects of α_2-adrenoreceptors on feeding rhythms across the diurnal cycle (Morien *et al.*, 1999; Diaz-Cabiale *et al.*, 2000). An infusion of oxytocin into the vagal complex in the medulla reduces intestinal mobility and stimulates the release of some gastrointestinal and pancreatic hormones via vagal pathways (Bitar *et al.*, 1980; Rogers and Herman, 1985; McCann and Rogers, 1990).

These findings suggest that during active labour, oxytocin operates via central and peripheral mechanisms to inhibit food intake and gastrointestinal activity. As labour progresses, cervical stretching and myometrial contractions stimulate uterine afferent nerve pathways to the hypothalamus stimulating both central and peripheral release of oxytocin (Antonijevic *et al.*, 1995). On the basis of current findings on the inhibitory effects of central oxytocin on food intake and gastrointestinal function, maternal food appetite can be expected to fall to non-existent levels during active labour. At the same time the powerful excitatory afferent pathways from the cervix to oxytocin cells in the hypothalamus may induce vomiting, particularly during the latter part of labour, which stimulates a reflexive dilatation of the cervix (Antonijevic *et al.*, 1995).

Energy requirements for myometrial contractions and maternal neocortical activity

At present, there is no research evidence to suggest that myometrial contractions impose additional demands on maternal energy stores during labour. Like all smooth muscle, the myometrium has been shown to have a low energy requirement and an increased capacity for glycogen storage. Under the influence of oestrogen and progesterone, myometrial glycogen stores increase up to tenfold during pregnancy, peak at term and are used as a predominant source of energy for contractions during and after labour (Brody, 1958; Wedenberg *et al.*, 1990; Steingrimsdottir *et al.*, 1993). At the same time, skeletal muscle activity tends to be minimized. It has also been suggested that maternal neocortical or higher brain requirements for glucose may also decline during labour, as women tend to withdraw and become remote from verbal communications around them (Odent, 1992, 1994; Keenan *et al.*, 1998).

Fetal responses to labour and birth

In the mature animal, the sympathoadrenal system functions to maintain homeostasis, in response to a wide variety of stressful stimuli, through activation of sympathetic nerve pathways and adrenomedullary secretions. These responses are largely controlled by the central nervous system through stimulation of splanchnic nerves that synapse with prevertebral ganglia in the spinal cord (Slotkin, 1990). In a number of species, including humans, chromaffin cells in the adrenal medulla and the abdominal aorta function independently of sympathetic innervation throughout gestation which gives them a unique capacity to respond directly to specific stressful stimuli (Phillippe, 1983; Slotkin, 1990). This developmental capacity persists until a few days following birth when the extra-adrenal islets of chromaffin cells start to degenerate and the adrenal medulla begins to acquire sympathetic innervation from the splanchnic nerves (Slotkin, 1990; Slotkin *et al.*, 1990).

The dominance of non-neurogenic catecholamine release in response to labour and birth seems to be part of a phased maturation of the stress axis in humans and other species. Before and after birth this selective response induces maturational changes in particular organ systems in preparation for extrauterine life while other well-defined stressors like hypoglycaemia do not evoke any adrenomedullary secretion (Slotkin, 1990; Widmaier, 1990). In the human fetus, catecholamine levels rise throughout labour, to reach 20 times adult resting values immediately following birth (Lagercrantz and Slotkin, 1986; Lagercrantz and Marcus, 1992). At the same time, free cortisol levels double in association with labour and rise further in the first hour or two following birth while a dramatic surge in thyrotrophin (TSH) at birth stimulates striking increases in thyroid hormones during the first 24 hours of neonatal life (Pearson Murphy and Branchaud, 1994; Girard and Pegorier, 1998).

Together, these neurohormonal stress responses regulate cardiorespiratory and metabolic adaptations to extrauterine life. TSH is the prime activator of lipolysis in white adipose tissue while catecholamines stimulate a sharp rise in plasma glucagon and a corresponding fall in plasma insulin (Marcus *et al.*, 1988). At the same time, experiments on lambs suggest that oxytocin has a significant stimulatory effect on glucagon, at plasma concentrations that occur during labour (Lawrence *et al.*, 1989). In the presence of low circulating levels of insulin and glucose, glucagon and adrenaline stimulate glycogenolysis while glucagon and long chain fatty acids (LCFAs) stimulate gene transcription of key enzymes involved in gluconeogenesis, lipolysis and ketogenesis throughout the suckling period (Pegorier *et al.*, 1998; Ktorza *et al.*, 1981; Martin *et al.*, 1981; Girard and Pegorier, 1998; Pegorier, 1998; Pegorier *et al.*, 1998).

Maternal HPA axis and oxytocin – influences on neonatal metabolic adaptations

The changes that occur in maternal food appetite and metabolism during active labour influence the transplacental supply of glucose, ketones and fatty acids until the moment of birth. Existing evidence suggests that the transition from carbohydrate to lipid metabolism in the neonate following birth is stimulated by transplacental supplies of ketones and fatty acids and inhibited by increased maternal glucose concentrations during labour (Ktorza et al., 1981; Martin et al., 1981; Girard et al., 1992; Chen et al., 1998). In humans, glucocorticoids and oxytocin may influence this transition through their opposing effects on maternal metabolism during active labour. In humans and other primates, basal levels of glucocorticoids begin to show a raised profile from approximately 25 weeks, in conjunction with adaptations in the hypothalamic-pituitary adrenocortical axis that seem to be stimulated by rising levels of oestrogen and a progressive decline in fasting glucose concentrations during the second half of pregnancy (Nolten and Rueck, 1981; Allolio et al., 1990; Goland et al., 1990, 1992; Widmaier, 1990; Vamvakopoulos and Chrousos, 1993).

Placental corticotrophin-releasing hormone (CRH)

In humans and other primates, placental CRH operates as part of maternal and fetal hypothalamic-pituitary-adrenal axes and is regulated by a positive feedback mechanism within the placenta (Pepe and Albrecht, 1995; Clifton et al., 1998; Leitch et al., 1998; McLean and Smith, 1999; Cheng et al., 2000). Longitudinal studies on women suggest that from around 15 weeks' gestation, placental CRH is released into the circulation and progressively increases by the end of pregnancy, to reach levels equivalent to those found in hypothalamic portal blood during stress (McLean et al., 1995; McLean and Smith, 1999). According to some but not all research findings, CRH activity is buffered by the presence of higher concentrations of CRH-binding protein (CRH-BP) until the last 3 weeks of pregnancy, when a rapid rise in plasma CRH is accompanied by a 50% fall in CRH-BP (Berkowitz *et al.*, 1996; McLean and Smith, 1999).

Current findings suggest that placental CRH operates through a number of receptor signalling pathways that have both stimulatory and inhibitory effects on myometrial contractility. In cultured myocytes before the onset of labour, CRH has been found to inhibit both basal and stimulated PGE_2 while oxytocin has been found to reduce the biological activity of CRH receptors that inhibit myometrial contractility (Grammatopoulos and Hillhouse, 1999a, 1999b; Grammatopoulos *et al.*, 1999). This finding suggests that as local oxytocin and oxytocin receptor expression increases at the end of pregnancy, a shift occurs from relaxation to regulated contractility which begins as a nocturnal event that coincides with the daily rhythm in plasma oxytocin concentrations (Fuchs *et al.*, 1992).

Hyporesponsiveness of the HPA axis to stress

In rodents, responsiveness of the hypothalamic-pituitary-adrenocortical axis (HPA) to physical and emotional stressors is progressively reduced from the latter part of pregnancy and during the entire period of parturition while a reduced stress response has been demonstrated in both rat and human studies during lactation (Franceschini *et al.*, 1989; Altemus *et al.*, 1995; Toufexis and Walker, 1996; Douglas *et al.*, 1998; Neumann *et al.*, 1998; Wigger *et al.*, 1999; Johnstone *et al.*, 2000). In rodents, the reduced HPA response to physical and emotional stressors in late pregnancy is activated at all levels of the axis, including reduced content of CRH mRNA in the paraventricular nucleus; reduced CRH responsiveness of pituitary corticotrophes and enhanced negative feedback of glucocorticoids (Johnstone *et al.*, 2000). In addition, central oxytocin seems to have an inhibitory effect on basal adrenocortico trophic hormone (ACTH) during late pregnancy while endogenous opioids tonically inhibit the HPA axis.

Consequently, plasma concentrations of ACTH and corticos-terone progressively decline in both rats and pigs during the entire process of parturition (Neumann *et al.*, 1998; Wigger *et al.*, 1999).

In humans and other primates, the progressive rise in pla-cental CRH is also accompanied by suppression of hypothal-amic CRH neurones and reduced anterior pituitary corti-cotrophin responses to CRH. Despite highly elevated levels of circulating CRH during the second half of pregnancy, ACTH remains within the normal range and no increase has been found in plasma ACTH in response to exogenous CRH during the third trimester (Schulte *et al.*, 1990; Goland *et al.*, 1990, 1992; Magiakon *et al.*, 1996). However, in humans evi-dence of an enhanced HPA axis has been found during labour, with significant increases in maternal ACTH and cor-tisol from late pregnancy through labour and birth (Carr *et al.*, 1981; Campbell *et al.*, 1987; Van Cauwenberge *et al.*, 1987; Chan *et al.*, 1993; Fajardo *et al.*, 1994; Ohana *et al.*, 1996; Chen *et al.*, 1998). In addition, emotional stress seems to be associ-ated with greater increases in maternal cortisol and glucose between late pregnancy and birth and higher concentrations of cortisol and glucose in cord blood immediately following birth (Chen *et al.*, 1998). Hormonal profiles on a small sample of women before and after labour have recently demon-strated increased levels of cortisol, lower concentrations of insulin and elevated serum glucose levels of around 6.8 mmol/l within the first hour following birth (Chen *et al.*, 1998). In this study, mean cord glucose concentrations were 5.92 mmol/l and this blood value emerged as the most pre-dictive of delayed lactogenesis (Chen *et al.*, 1998).

These findings suggest that emotional stress during labour is associated with increased HPA activity and cortisol induced hyperglycaemia that seems to have negative implications for the shift from carbohydrate to lipid metabolism in the neonate (Martin *et al.*, 1981). From late pregnancy onwards, central oxytocin may counter this effect, through its capacity to modulate the HPA axis by ameliorating anxiety. During active labour and birth, central oxytocin may also reduce maternal glucose levels by inhibiting maternal appetite while the pulsatile release of oxytocin may reduce glucose concentrations by stimulating glucose transport, oxidation and lipogenesis and by inhibiting catecholamine-stimulated lipolysis in maternal adipose tissue.

Conclusion

From early pregnancy onwards changes occur in maternal appetite, gastrointestinal functions and metabolism that seem to anticipate the distinct developmental needs of the embryo, fetus and neonate. During the highly sensitive period of embryonic formation, episodes of hunger, nausea and vomiting coincide with heightened anabolism, as maternal adipose tissue is laid down in preparation for rapid growth during fetal and neonatal development. Following the period of rapid fetal growth between 18 and 34 weeks' gestation, the earlier maternal tendency to accumulate adipose tissue diminishes and stores begin to decline, as enhanced adipose tissue lipolysis becomes a characteristic feature of *both* fed and fasted states.

When fetal growth slows down from around 36 weeks' gestation, maternal adipose tissue begins to decline, as increased placental uptake of nutrients is accompanied by increased storage of lipids by the mammary gland, in preparation for milk synthesis during lactation. During the final weeks of pregnancy and the early phases of labour, heightened secretion of PRL may increase maternal appetite while circulating lipid concentrations decline; glucose tolerance improves and glucose stimulated insulin secretion declines. Once active labour begins, increased oxytocin secretion reduces maternal food appetite and gastrointestinal motility and in the absence of stress-induced activation of cortisol, glucose remains at fasting concentrations. Along with the stress-induced activation of glucagon and the inhibition of insulin secretion at birth, low maternal glucose levels during active labour facilitate the enzymatic changes that regulate the transition from carbohydrate to lipid metabolism and the shift from placental to mammary nutrition.

References

Ahima, R.S., Saper, C., Flier, J.S. and Elmquist, J.K. (2000) Leptin regulation of neuroendocrine systems. *Frontiers in Neuroendocrinology* 21: 263–307

Allolio, B., Hoffmann, J., Linton, E.A., Winkelmann, W., Kusche, M. and Schulte, H.M. (1990) Diurnal salivary cortisol patterns during pregnancy and after delivery: relationship to plasma corticotrophin-releasing hormone. *Clinical Endocrinology* 33: 279–89

Alsat, E., Guibourdenche, J., Lutton, D., Frankenne, F. and Evian-Brion, D. (1997) Human placental growth hormone. *American Journal of Obstetrics and Gynecology* 177 (6): 1526–34

Altemus, M., Deuster, P.A., Galliven, E., Carter, C.S. and Gold, P.W. (1995) Suppression of hypothalamic–pituitary–adrenal axis responses to stress in lactating women. *Journal of Clinical Endocrinology and Metabolism* 80 (10): 2954–9

Altszuler, N. and Fuchs, A-R. (1994) Oxytocin secretion is stimulated by changes in glucose metabolism. *Proceedings of the Society for Experimental Biology and Medicine* 207: 38–42

Altszuler, N. and Hampshire, J. (1981) Oxytocin infusion increases plasma insulin and glucagon levels and glucose production and uptake in the normal dog. *Diabetes* 30: 112–14

Altszuler, N., Rosenberg, C.R., Winkler, B., Fuchs, A.R., Hill, P.S. and Hruby, V.J. (1992)The metabolic effects of oxytocin are mediated by a uterine type receptor and are inhibited by oxytocin antagonist and by arginine vasopressin in the dog. *Life Science* 50: 739–46

Antonijevic, I.A., Leng, G., Luckman. S.M., Douglas, A.J., Bicknell, R.J. and Russell, J.A. (1995) Induction of uterine activity with oxytocin in late pregnant rats replicates the expression of *c-fos* in neuroendocrine and brain stem neurones as seen during parturition. *Endocrinology* 136 (1): 154–63

Arletti, R., Benelli, A. and Bertolini, A. (1989) Influence of oxytocin on feeding behaviour in the rat. *Peptides* 10: 89–93

Baird, J.D. (1986) Some aspects of the metabolic and hormonal adaptation to pregnancy. *Acta Endocrinologica, Supplementum* 277: 11–18

Bandyopadhyay, G.K., Lee, L-Y., Guzman, R.C. and Nandi, S. (1995) Effect of reproductive states on lipid mobilization and linoleic acid metabolism in mammary glands. *Lipids* 30 (2): 155–62

Barash, V. *et al.* (1983) Mechanism of placental glycogen deposition in diabetes in the rat. *Diabetologia* 24: 63

Barrett, J.F.R., Whittaker, P.G., Williams, J.G. and Lind, T. (1994) Absorption of non-haem iron from food during normal pregnancy. *British Medical Journal* 309: 79–82

Battaglia, F.C. (1978) Commonality and diversity in fetal development: bridging the interspecies gap. *Pediatric Research* 12: 736–42

Beaudry, M.A., Chiasson, J.L. and Exton, J.H. (1977) Gluconeogenesis in the suckling rat. *American Journal of Physiology* 233 (2): E175–E180

Berkowitz, G.S., Lapinski, R.H., Lockwood, C.J., Florio, P., Blackmore-Prince, C. and Petraglia, F. (1996) Corticotrophin-releasing factor and its binding protein: maternal serum levels in term and preterm deliveries. *American Journal of Obstetrics and Gynecology* 174: 1477–83

Besnard, P., Foucaud, L., Mallordy, A., Berges, C., Kaikaus, R.M., Bernard, A. *et al.* (1995) Expression of fatty acid binding protein in the liver during pregnancy and lactation in the rat. *Biochemica et Biophysica Acta* 1258: 153–8

Bispham, J., Heasman, L., Clarke, L., Ingleton, P.M., Stephenson, T. and Symonds, M.E. (1999) Effect of maternal dexamethasone treatment and ambient temperature on pro-lactin receptor abundance in brown adipose and hepatic tissue in the foetus and new-born lamb. *Journal of Neuroendocrinology* 11: 849–56

Bitar, K.N., Said, S.L., Weir, G.C., Saffouri, B. and Makhlouf, G.M. (1980) Neural release of vasoactive intestinal peptide from the gut. *Gastroenterology* 79: 1288–94

Bjorkstrand, E. and Uvnas-Moberg, K. (1996) Central oxy-tocin increases food intake and daily weight gain in rats. *Physiology and Behaviour* 59 (4/5): 947–52

Bjorkstrand, E., Eriksson, M. and Uvnas-Moberg, K. (1992) Plasma levels of oxytocin after food deprivation and hypo-glycaemia, and effects of 1-deamino-2-D-Tyr-(OEt)-4-Thr-8-Orn-oxytocin on blood glucose in rats. *Acta Physiologica Scandinavica* 144: 355–9

Bjorkstrand, E., Eriksson, M. and Uvnas-Moberg, K. (1996) Evidence of a peripheral and a central effect of oxytocin on pan-creatic hormone release in rats. *Neuroendocrinology*, 63: 377–83

Blackburn, R.E., Demko, A.D., Hoffman, G.E., Stricker, E.M. and Verbalis, J.G. (1992) Central oxytocin inhibition of angiotensin-induced salt appetite in rats. *American Journal of Physiology* 263 (32): R1347–R53

Bougneres, P.F., Lemmel, C., Ferre, P. and Bier, D.M. (1986) Ketone body transport in the neonate and infant. *Journal of Clinical Investigation* 77: 42–8

Bozzetti, P., Ferrari, M.M., Marconi, A.M., Ferrazzi, E., Pardi, G., Makowski, E.L. *et al.* (1988) The relationship of maternal and fetal glucose concentration from mid-gestation until term. *Metabolism* 37 (4): 358–63

Brelje, C.T. and Sorenson, R.L. (1991) Role of prolactin versus growth hormone on islet β–cell proliferation in vitro: implications for pregnancy. *Endocrinology* 128: 45–57

Brelje, C.T., Parsons, J.A. and Sorenson, R.L. (1994) Regulation of islet β-cell proliferation by prolactin in rat islets. *Diabetes* 43: 263–73

Brelje, C.T., Scharp, D.W., Lacy, P.E., Ogren, L., Talamantes, F., Robertson, M., Friesen, H.G. and Sorenson, R.L. (1993) Effect of homologous placental lactogens, prolactins, and growth hormones on islet β-cell division and insulin secretion in rat, mouse, and human islets: implications for placental lactogen regulation of islet function during pregnancy. *Endocrinogy* 132 (2): 879–87

Brenton, C., Pechoux, C., Morel, G. and Zingg, H.H. (1995) Oxytocin receptor messenger ribonucleic acid: characterisation, regulation, and cellular localization in the rat pituitary gland. *Endocrinology* 136 (7): 2928–36

Briski, K.P. and Brandt, J.A. (2000) Oxytocin and vasopressin neurones in principal and accessory hypothalamic magnocellular structures express *Fos*-immunoreactivity in response to acute glucose deprivation. *Journal of Neuroendocrinology* 12: 409–14

Brody, S. (1958) Hormonal influence on the glycogen content of the human myometrium. *Acta Endocrinologica* 27: 377–84

Bull, P.M., Douglas, A.J. and Russell, J.A. (1994) Opioids and coupling of the anterior peri-third ventricular input to oxytocin neurones in anaesthetized pregnant rats. *Journal of Neuroendocrinology* 6: 267–74

Byatt, J.C., Staten, N.R., Salgiver, W.J., Kostelc, J.G. and Collier, R.J. (1993) Stimulation of food intake and weight gain in mature female rats by bovine prolactin and bovine growth hormone. *American Journal of Physiology* 264 (27): E986–E92

Campbell, E.A., Linton, E.A., Wolfe, C.D.A., Scraggs, P.R., Jones, M.T., and Lowry, P.J. (1987) Plasma corticotrophin-releasing hormone concentrations during pregnancy and parturition. *Journal of Clinical Endocrinology and Metabolism* 64 (5): 1054–9

Campbell, F.M., Gordon, M.J. and Dutta-Roy, A.K. (1996) Preferential uptake of long chain polyunsaturated fatty acids by isolated human placental membranes. *Molecular and Cellular Biochemistry* 155: 77–83

Carr, B.R.., Parker, C.R., Madden, J.D., MacDonald, P.C. and Porter, J.C. (1981) Maternal plasma adrenocorticotrophin and cortisol relationships throughout pregnancy. *American Journal of Obstetrics and Gynecology* 139 (4): 416–22

Caruso, A., Paradisi, G., Ferrazani Slucchese, A., Moretti, S. and Fulghesu, A.M. (1998) Effect of maternal carbohydrate metabolism on fetal growth. *Obstetrics and Gynaecology* 92 (1): 8–12

Casanueva, F.F. and Diguez, C. (1999) Neuroeodocrine regulation and actions of leptin. *Frontiers in Neuroendocrinology* 20: 317–63

Chaffin, D.G., Clark, R.M., McCracken, D. and Phillips, A.F. (1995) Effect of hypoinsulinemia on growth in the fetal rabbit. *Biology of the Neonate* 67: 186–93

Chan, E-C., Smith, R., Lewin, T. *et al.* (1993) Plasma corticotrophin-releasing hormone, β-endorphin and cortisol interrelationships during human pregnancy. *Acta Endocrinologica* 128: 339–44

Chen, D.C., Nommsen-Rivers, L., Dewey, K.G. and Lonnerdal, B. (1998) Stress during labour and delivery and early lactation performance. *American Journal of Clinical Nutrition* 68: 335–44

Chez, R.A., Mintz, D.H., Epstein, M.R., Fleischman, A.R., Oakes, G.K. and Dutchinson, D.L. (1974) Glucagon metabolism in non human primate pregnancy. *American Journal of Obstetrics and Gynecology*, 120: 690–6

Cheng, Y-H., Nicholson, R.C., King, B., Chan, E-C., Fitter, J.T. and Smith, R. (2000) Glucocorticoid stimulation of corticotrophin-releasing hormone gene expression requires a cyclic adenosine 3′,5′-monophosphate regulatory element in human primary placental cytotrophoblast cells. *Journal of Clinical Endocrinology and Metabolism* 85 (5): 1937–45

Chiodera, P., Volpi, R., Capretti, L., Speroni, G., Marcato, A., Rossi, G. and Coiro, V. (1992) Hypoglycaemia-induced arginine vasopressin and oxytocin release is mediated by glucoreceptors located inside the blood–brain barrier. *Neuroendocrinology* 55: 655–9

Clandinin, M.T. (1999) Brain development and assessing the supply of polyunsaturated fatty acid. *Lipids* 34 (2): 131–7

Clifton, V.L., Telfer, J.F., Thompson, A.J., Cameron, I.T., Teoh, T.G., Lye, S.J. and Challis, J.R.J. (1998) Corticotrophin-releasing hormone and proopiomelanocortin-derived peptides are present in human myometrium. *Journal of Clinical Endocrinology and Metabolism* 83 (10): 3716–21

Condliffe, S.B., Doolan, C.M. and Harvey, B.J. (2001) 17β-oestradiol acutely regulates CL⁻ secretion in rat distal colonic epithelium. *Journal of Physiology* 530 (1): 47–54

Coskun, T., Bozkurt, A., Alican, I., Ozkutlu, U., Kurtel, H. and Yegen, C. (1997) Pathways mediating CRF-induced inhibition of gastric emptying in rats. *Regulatory Peptides* 69: 113–20

Crawford, J.S. (1956) Some aspects of obstetric anaesthesia. *British Journal of Anaesthesia* 28: 201–8

Crowley, R.S., Insel, T.R., O'Keefe, J.A. and Amico, J.A. (1995) Increased accumulation of oxytocin messenger ribonucleic acid in the hypothalamus of the female rat: induction by long term estradiol and progesterone administration and subsequent progesterone withdrawal. *Endocrinology,* 136 (1): 224–31

Da Costa, T.H.M. and Williamson, D.H. (1994) Regulation of rat mammary-gland uptake of orally admininstered [1-^{14}C] triolein by insulin and prolactin: evidence for bihormonal control of lipoprotein lipase activity. *Biochemistry Journal* 300: 257–62

Dahlquist, G., Persson, U. and Persson, B. (1972) The activity of *D*-β-hydroxybutyrate dehydrogenase in fetal, infant and adult rat brain and the influence of starvation. *Biology of the Neonate* 20: 40–50

Darmady, J. and Postle, A.D. (1982) Lipid metabolism in pregnancy. *British Journal of Obstetrics and Gynaecology* 89: 211–215

Devaskar, S.U., Ganguli, S., Styer, D., Devaskar, U.P. and Sperling, M.A. (1984) Glucagon and glucose dynamics in sheep: evidence for glucagon resistance in the fetus. *American Journal of Physiology,* 246: 256–65

Diaz-Cabiale, Z., Narvaez, J.A., Petersson, M., Uvnas-Moberg, K. and Fuxe, K. (2000) Oxytocin/alpha$_2$-adrenoceptor interactions in feeding responses. *Neuroendocrinology* 71: 209–18

Dobbing, J. and Sands, J. (1973) Quantitiative growth and development of human brain. *Archives of Diseases in Childhood* 48: 757–67

Douglas, A.J., Johnstone, H.A., Wigger, A., Landgraf, R. and Russell, J.A. (1998) The role of endogenous opioids in neuro-hypophysial and hypothalamic–pituitary–adrenal axis hormone secretory responses to stress in pregnant rats. *Journal of Endocrinology,* 158: 285–93

Dutta-Roy, A.K. (1997) Fatty acid transport and metabolism in the feto-placental unit and the role of the fatty acid-binding proteins. *Nutritional Biochemistry* 8: 548–57

Elkington, K.W. (1991) At the water's edge: where obstetrics and anaesthesia meet. *Obstetrics and Gynaecology* 77 (2): 304–8

Elliot, J.A. (1975) The effect of pregnancy on the control of lipolysis in fat cells isolated from human adipose tissue. *European Journal Clinical Investigation,* 5: 159–63

Emond, M., Ladenheim, E.E., Schwartz, G.J. and Moran, T.H. (2001) Leptin amplifies the feeding inhibition and neural activation arising from a gastric nutrient preload. *Physiology and Behaviour* 72: 123–8

Eriksson, L., Frankenne, F., Eden, S., Hennen, G. and Von Schoultz, B. (1989) Growth hormone 24h serum profile during pregnancy – lack of pulsatility for the secretion of the placental variant. *British Journal of Obstetrics and Gynaecology* 96: 949–53

Fajardo, M.C., Florido, J., Villaverde, C., Oltras, C.M., Gonzalez-Ramirez, A.R. and Gonzalez-Gomez, F. (1994) *European Journal of Obstetrics and Gynaecology* 55: 105–8

Feldman, M., Van Aerde, J.E. and Clandinin, M.T. (1992) Lipid accretion in the fetus and newborn. In Polin, R.A. and Fox, W.W. (eds), *Fetal and Neonatal Physiology.* Philadelphia: WB Saunders, pp. 299–31

Fielder, P.J. and Talamantes, F. (1987) The lipolytic effects of mouse placental lactogen II, mouse prolactin, mouse growth hormone, on adipose tissue from virgin and pregnant mice. *Endocrinology* 121: 493–7

Fisher, B.M., Bayliss, P.H. and Frier, B.M. (1987) Plasma oxytocin, arginine, vasopressin and atrial natriuretic peptide responses to insulin-induced hypoglycaemia in man. *Clinical Endocrinology* 26: 179–85

Flanagan, L.M., Olson, B.R., Sved, A.F., Verbalis, J.G. and Stricker, E.M. (1992) Gastric motility in conscious rats given oxytocin and oxytocin antagonist centrally. *Brain Research* 578: 356–60

Flanagan-Cato, L.M., King, J.K., Blechman, J.G. and O'Brien, M.P. (1998) Estrogen reduces cholecystokinin-induced *c-fos* expression in the rat brain. *Neuroendocrinology* 67: 384–91

Fleenor, D., Petryk, A., Driscoll, P. and Freemark, M. (2000) Constitutive expression of placental lactogen in pancreatic beta cells: effects on cell morphology, growth and gene expression. *Pediatric Research* 47: 136–142

Flint, D.J., Sinnett-Smith, P.A., Clegg, R.A. and Vernon, R.G. (1979) Role of insulin receptors in the changing metabolism of adipose tissue during pregnancy and lactation in the rat. *Biochemistry Journal* 182: 421–9

Fowden, A.L. (1989) The role of insulin in prenatal growth. *Journal of Developmental Physiology* 12: 173–82

Fowden, A.L., Forhead, A.J., Bloomfield, M., Taylor, P.M. and Silver, M. (1999) Pancreatic *a* cell function in the fetal foal during late gestation. *Experimental Physiology* 84: 697–705

Franceschini, R. *et al.* (1989) Plasma beta-endorphin concentration during suckling in lactating women. *British Journal of Obstetrics and Gynaecology*, 96: 711–13

Frankenne, F., Closset, J., Gomez, F., Scippo, M.L., Smal, J. and Hennen, G. (1988) The physiology of growth hormone (GHs) in pregnant women and partial characterisation of the placental GH variant. *Journal of Clinical Endocrinology and Metabolism* 66 (6): 1171–80

Frankenne, F., Scippo, M-L., Beeumen, J.V., Igout, A. and Hennen, G. (1990) Identification of placental human growth hormone as the growth hormone-V gene expression product. *Journal of Clinical Endocrinology and Metabolism* 71 (1): 15–18

Frankenne, F., Closset, J., Gomez, F., Scippo, M.L., Smal, J., Hennen, G. (1988) The physiology of growth hormones (GHs) in pregnant women and partial characterisation of the placental GH variant. *Journal of Clinical Endocrinology and Metabolism* 66 (6): 1171–80.

Fraser, R.B. (1991) Carbohydrate metabolism. In Hytten, F. and Chamberlain, G. (eds), *Clinical Physiology in Obstetrics*. Oxford: Blackwell Scientific, pp. 204–12

Freemark, M. (1999a) Editorial: The fetal adrenal and the maturation of the growth hormone and prolactin axes. *Endocrinology* 140 (5): 1963–5

Freemark, M. (1999b) The role of growth hormone, prolactin, and placental lactogen in human fetal development. In Handwerger, S. (ed.), *Molecular and Cellular Pediatric Endocrinology*. Totowa, NJ: Humana Press, pp. 57–83

Freemark, M., Fleenor, D., Driscoll, P., Binark, N. and Kelly, P.A. (2001) Body weight and fat deposition in prolactin receptor-deficient mice. *Endocrinology* 142 (2): 532–7

Freinkel, N. (1980) Of pregnancy and pogen. *Diabetes* 29: 1023–33

Fuchs, A-R., Romero, R., Keefe, D., Parra, M., Oyarzun, E. and Behnke, E. (1991) Oxytocin secretion and human parturition: pulse frequency and duration increase during spontaneous labour. *American Journal of Obstetrics and Gynecology*, 165 (5): 1515–23

Fuchs, A-R., Behrens, O. and Liu, H–C. (1992) Correlation of nocturnal increase in plasma oxytocin with a decrease in plasma estradiol/progesterone ratio in late pregnancy. *American Journal of Obstetrics and Gynecology* 167 (6): 1559–63

Gao, Z-Y., Drews, G. and Henquin, J–C. (1991) Mechanisms of the stimulation of insulin release by oxytocin in normal mouse islets. *Biochemistry Journal* 276: 169–74

Gerardo-Gettens, T., Moore, B.J., Stern, J.S. and Horwitz, B.A. (1989) Prolactin stimulates food intake in a dose-dependent matter. *American Journal of Physiology* 256 (25): R276–80

Ghebremeskel, K., Bitsanis, D., Koukkou, E., Lowy, C., Poston, L. and Crawford, M.A. (1999) Maternal diet high in fat reduces docosahexanic acid in liver lipids of newborn and suckling rat pups. *British Journal of Nutrition* 81: 395–404

Gimpl, G. and Farenholz, F. (2001) The oxytocin receptor system: structure, function, and regulation. *Physiological Reviews* 81 (2): 629–83

Girard, G.R. (1975) Metabolic fuels of the fetus. *Israeli Journal of Medical Science* 11 (6): 591–600

Girard, J. and Pegorier, J-P. (1998) An overview of early post-partum nutrition and metabolism. *Biochemical Society Transactions* 26: 69–74

Girard, J., Ferre, P., Pegorier, J-P. and Duee, P-H. (1992) Adaptations of glucose and fatty acid metabolism during perinatal period and suckling–weaning transition. *Physiological Reviews* 72 (2): 507–62

Girard, G.R., Kervran, A., Soufflet, E. and Assan, R. (1974) Factors affecting the secretion of insulin and glucagon by the rat fetus. *Diabetes* 23: 310–17

Godfrey Robinson, S.K.M., Barker, D.J.P., Osmond, C. and Cox, V. (1996) Maternal nutrition in early and late pregnancy in relation to placental and fetal growth. *British Medical Journal*, 312: 410–14

Goland, R.S., Conwell, I.M., Warren, W.B. *et al.* (1992) Placental corticotrophin-releasing hormone and pituitary–adrenal function during pregnancy. *Neuroendocrinology* 56: 742–9

Goland, R.S., Stark, R.I. and Wardlaw, S.L. (1990) Responses to corticotrophin-releasing hormone during pregnancy in the baboon. *Journal of Clinical Endocrinology and Metabolism* 70 (4): 925–29

Golde, S.H., Good-Anderson, B., Montro, M. and Artal, R. (1982) Insulin requirements during labour: A reappraisal. *American Journal of Obstetrics and Gynecology* 144 (5): 556–9

Goluboff, L. and Ezrin, C. (1969) Effects of pregnancy on the somatotroph and the prolactin cell of the human adenohypophysis. *Journal of Clinical Endocrinology and Metabolism*, 29: 1533–8

Goodman, H.M. and Coiro, V. (1981) Induction of sensitivity to insulin-like action of growth hormone in normal rat adipose tissue. *Endocrinology* 108 (1): 113–19

Goodman, H.M. and Grichting, G. (1983) Growth hormone and lipolysis: a reevaluation. *Endocrinology* 113 (5): 1697–702

Goodman, H.M., Tai, L-R., Ray, J., Cooke, N.E. and Liebhaber, S.A. (1991) Human growth hormone variant produces insulin-like and lipolytic responses in rat adipose tissue. *Endocrinology* 129 (4): 1779–83

Grammatopoulos, D.K. and Hillhouse, E.W. (1999a) Activation of protein kinase C by oxytocin inhibits the biological activity of the human myometrial corticotrophin-releasing hormone receptor at term. *Endocrinology* 140: 585–94

Grammatopoulos, D.K. and Hillhouse, E.W. (1999b) Basal and interleukin-1β-stimulated prostaglandin production from cultured human myometrial cells: differential regulation by corticotrophin-releasing hormone. *Journal of Clinical Endocrinology and Metabolism* 84: 2204–11

Grammatopoulos, D.K., Dai, Y. and Randeva, H.S. (1999) Role of corticotrophin-releasing hormone in onset of labour. *Lancet* 354: 1546–9

Gustafson, A.B., Banasiak, M.F., Kalkhoff, R.K., Hagen, T.C. and Kim, H. (1980) Correlation of hyperprolactinaemia with altered plasma insulin and glucagon: Similarity to effects of late human pregnancy. *Journal of Clinical Endocrinology and Metabolism* 51: 242–6

Haanwinckel, M.A., Ellias, L.K., Favaretto, A.L.V., Gutkowska, J. and McCann, S.M. (1995) Oxytocin mediates atrial natriuetoic peptide release and natriuresis after volume expansion in the rat. *Proceedings National Academy Science* 92: 7902–6

Haggarty, P., Ashton, J., Johnson, M. and Abramovich, D.R. (1999) Effect of maternal polyunsaturated fatty acid concentration on transport by the human placenta. *Biology of the Neonate* 75: 350–9

Haggarty, P., Page, K., Abramovich, D.R., Ashton, J. and Brown, D. (1997) Long-chain polyunsaturated fatty acid transport across the perfused human placenta. *Placenta* 18: 635–42

Hanif, K., Goren, H.J., Hollenberg, M.D. and Lederis, K. (1982) Oxytocin action: mechanisms for insulin-like activity in isolated rat adipocytes. *Molecular Pharmacology* 22: 381–8

Harding, J.E. and Evans, P.C. (1991) β-hydroxybutyrate is an alternative substrate for the fetal sheep brain. *Journal of Developmental Physiology* 16: 29–39

Hay, W.W. (1995) Metabolic interrelationships of placenta and fetus. *Placenta* 16: 19–30

Hay-Schmidt, A., Helboe, L. and Larsen, P.J. (2001) Leptin receptor immunoreactivity is present in ascending serotonergic and catecholaminergic neurones of the rat. *Neuroendocrinology* 73: 215–26

Heil, S.H. (1999) Sex-specific effects of prolactin on food intake by rats. *Hormones and Behaviour* 35: 47–54

Heim, T. (1983) Energy and lipid requirements of the fetus and the preterm infant. *Journal of Pediatric Gastroenterology and Nutrition* 2 (Suppl 1): S16–18

Heinrichs, S.C. and Richards, D.(1999) The role of corticotrophin-releasing factor and urocortin in the modulation of ingestive behaviour. *Neuropeptides* 33 (5): 350–9

Herrera, E. (2000) Metabolic adaptations in pregnancy and their implications for the availability of substrates to the fetus. *European Journal of Clinical Nutrition* 54 (Supplement 1): S47–S51

Herrera, E. and Amudquivar, E. (2000) Lipid metabolism in the fetus and the neonate. *Diabetes/Metabolism Research and Reviews* 16: 202–10

Herrera, E., Gomez-Coronodo, D. and Lasuncion, M.A. (1987) Lipid metabolism in pregnancy. *Biology of the Neonate* 51: 70–7

Herrera, E., Lasuncion, M.A., Gomez-Coronado, D., Aranda, P., Lopez-Luna, P. and Maier, I. (1988) Role of lipoprotein lipase activity on lipoprotein metabolism and the fate of circulating triglycerides in pregnancy. *American Journal of Obstetrics and Gynecology* 158 (6): 1575–83

Herrera, E., Lasuncion, M.A., Gomez-Coranado, L., Martin, A. and Bonet, B. (1990) Lipid metabolic interactions in the mother during pregnancy and their fetal repercussions. In Cuezva, J.M., Pascual-Leon, A.M. and Patel, M.S. (eds), *Endocrine and Biochemical Development of the Fetus and Neonate.* New York: Plenum Press, pp. 213–30

Herrera, E., Lasuncion, M.A. and Asuncion, M. (1992) Placental transport of free fatty acids, glycerol, and ketone bodies. In Polin, R.A. and Fox, W.W. (eds), *Fetal and Neonatal Physiology.* Philadelphia: WB Saunders. pp. 291–8

Hervey, G. (1969) Regulation of energy balance. *Nature* 222: 629–31

Hill, D.J. and Milner, R.D.G. (1985) Insulin as a growth factor. *Pediatric Research* 19 (9): 879–86

Hill, D.J., Strutt, B., Arny, E., Zaina, S., Coukell, S. and Graham, C.F. (2000) Increased and persistent circulating insulin–like growth factor II in neonatal transgenic mice suppresses developmental aptosis in the pancreatic islets. *Endocrinology* 141 (3): 1151–7

Holness, M.J., Munns, M.J. and Sugden, M.C. (1999) Current

concepts concerning the role of leptin in reproductive function. *Molecular and Cellular Endocrinology*, 157: 11–20

Hornnes, P.J. and Kuhl, C. (1986) Gastrointestinal hormones and cortisol in normal pregnant women and women with gestational diabetes. *Acta Endocrinologica Supplementum* 277: S24–S30

Hornstra, G. (2000) Essential fatty acids in mothers and their neonates. *American Journal of Clinical Nutrition*, 71 (Suppl): 1262S–9S

Huxley, R.R. (2000) Nausea and vomiting in early pregnancy: its role in placental development. *Obstetrics and Gynaecology* 95 (5): 779–82

Hytten, F.E. (1980) The alimentary system. In Hytten, F.E. and Chamberlain, G. (eds), *Clinical Physiology in Obstetrics*. Oxford: Blackwell Scientific, pp. 147–62

Igal, R.A., de Gomez Dumm, I.N.T. and Goya, R.G. (1998) Modulation of rat liver lipid metabolism by prolactin. *Prostaglandins*, *Leucotrienes and Essential Fatty Acids* 59 (6): 395–400

Innis, S.M. (1991) Essential fatty acids in growth and development. *Lipid Research* 30: 39–103

Jirikowski, G.F., Caldwell, J.D., Pilgrim, C., Stumpf, W.E. and Pedersen, C.A. (1989) Changes in immunostaining for oxytocin in the forebrain of the female rat during late pregnancy, parturition and early lactation. *Cell Tissue Research* 256: 411–17

Johnstone, H.A., Wigger, A., Douglas, A.J., Neumann, I.D., Landgraf, R., Seckl, J.R. and Russell, J.A. (2000) Attenuation of hypothalamic–pituitary–adrenal axis stress responses in late pregnancy: changes in feedforward and feedback mechanisms. *Journal of Neuroendocrinology* 12: 811–22

Jones, C.T. (1976) Lipid metabolism and mobilization in the guinea pig during pregnancy. *Biochemistry Journal* 156: 357–65

Jovanovic, L. and Perterson, C.M. (1983) Insulin and glucose requirements during the first stage of labour in insulin-dependent diabetic women. *American Journal of Medicine* 75: 607–12

Kalra, S.P., Dube, M.G., Pu, S., Xu, B. and Horvath, T.L. (1999) Integrating appetite-regulating pathways in the hypothalamic regulation of body weight. *Endocrine Reviews* 20 (1): 68–100

Kaneta, M., Edward, A., Liechty, H.C., Moorhead, H.C. and Lemons, J.A. (1991) Ovine fetal and maternal glycogen during fasting. *Biology of the Neonate* 60: 215–20

Kaplan, S.A. (1981) The insulin receptor. *Pediatric Research* 15: 1156–62

Kassem, S.A., Ariel, L., Thornton, P.S., Scheimberg, I. and Glaser, B. (2000) β-cell proliferation in the developing normal human pancreas and in hyperinsulinism of infancy. *Diabetes* 49: 1325–33

Keenan, P.A., Yaldoo, D.T., Stress, M.E., Fuerst, D.R., Ginsburg, K.A. *et al.* (1998) Explicit memory in pregnant women. *American Journal of Obstetrics and Gynecology* 179 (3): 731–7

Kern, W., Schiefer, B., Schwarzenburg, J., Stange, E.F., Born, J. and Fehm, H.L. (1997) Evidence for central nervous effects of corticotrophin-releasing hormone on gastric acid secretion in humans. *Neuroendocrinology* 65: 291–8

Knopp, R.H., Herrera, E. and Frenkel, N. (1970) Carbohydrate metabolism in pregnancy: VIII. Metabolism of adipose tissue isolated from fed and fasted pregnant rats during late gestation. *Journal of Clinical Investigation*, 49: 1438–46

Knopp, R.H., Montes, A., Childs, M., Job, R. and Mabuchi, H. (1981) Metabolic adjustments in normal and diabetic pregnancy. *Clinical Obstetrics and Gynaecology* 24 (1): 21–49

Knudtzon, J. (1983) Acute effects of oxytocin and vasopressin in plasma levels of glucagon, insulin and glucose in rabbits. *Hormone Metabolism Research* 15: 103–4

Kojima, M., Hosoda, H., Date, Y., Nakazato, M., Matsuo, H. and Kangawa, K. (1999) Ghrelin is a growth-hormone-releasing acylated peptide from stomach. *Nature* 402: 656–60

Kokkotou, E.G., Tritos, N.A., Mastaitis, J.W., Slieker, L. and Maratos-Flier, E. (2001) Melanin-concentrating hormone receptor is a target of leptin action in the mouse brain. *Endocrinology* 142 (2): 680–6

Kovacs, C.S. and Kronenberg, H.M. (1997) Maternal-fetal calcium and bone metabolism during pregnancy, puerperium, and lactation. *Endocrine Reviews* 18 (6): 832–72

Krahn, D.D., Gosnell, B.A., Grace, M. and Levine, A.S. (1986) CRF antagonist partially reverses CRF and stress–induced effects on feeding. *Brain Research Bulletin* 17: 285

Ktorza, A., Bihoreau, M-T., Nurjhan, N., Picon, L. and Girard, J. (1985) Insulin and glucagon during the perinatal period: secretion and metabolic effects on the liver. *Biology of the Neonate* 48: 204–20

Ktorza, A., Girard, J., Kinebanyan, M.F. and Picon, L. (1981) Hyperglycaemia induced by glucose infusion in unrestrained pregnant rat during the last 3 days of gestation: metabolic and hormonal changes in the mother and the fetus. *Diabetologia* 21: 569–74

Kubota, T., Kamada, S. and Saito, M. (1988) Prolactin-releasing system in the hypothalamo-pituitary axis in human early puerperium. In Mizuno, Mori and Taketani (eds), *Role of Prolactin in Human Reproduction*. Karger: Basle, pp. 253–63

Lacroix, R., Eason, E. and Melzack, R. (2000) Nausea and vomiting during pregnancy: a prospective study of its frequency, intensity, and patterns of change. *American Journal of Obstetrics and Gynecology* 182 (4): 931–7

Lagercrantz, H. and Marcus, C. (1992) Sympathoadrenal mechanisms during development. In Polin, R.A. and Fox, W.W. (eds), *Fetal and Neonatal Physiology.* Philadelphia: WB Saunders, pp. 160–9

Lagercrantz, H. and Slotkin, T.A. (1986) The 'stress' of being born. *Scientific American* 254: 92–102

Lambillotte, C., Gilon, P. and Henquin, J-C. (1997) Direct glucocorticcoid inhibition of insulin secretion. *Journal of Clinical Investigation* 9 (3): 414–23

Langhoff-Roos, J., Wibell, L., Gebre-Medhin, M. and Lindmark, G. (1989) Placental hormones and maternal glucose metabolism. A study of fetal growth in normal pregnancy. *British Journal of Obstetrics and Gynaecology*, 96: 320–6

Lawrence, A., Wallin, C., Fawcett, P. and Rosenfeld, C.R. (1989) Oxytocin stimulates glucagon and insulin secretion in fetal and neonatal sheep. *Endocrinology* 125 (5): 2289–96

Lawson, M., Kern, F. and Everson, G.T. (1985) Gastrointestinal transit time in human pregnancy: prolongation in the second and third trimesters followed by postpartum normalization. *Gastroenterology* 89: 996–1000

Leitch, I.M., Boura, A.L.A., Botti, C., Read, M.A., Walters, W.A.W. and Smith, R. (1998) Vasodilator actions of urocortin and related peptides in the human perfused placenta *in vitro*. *Journal of Clinical Endocrinology and Metabolism* 83 (12): 4510–13

Leng, G. and Brown, D. (1997) The origins and significance of pulsatility in hormone secretion from the pituitary. *Journal of Neuroendocrinology* 9: 493–513

Leng, G., Brown, C.H. and Russell, J.A. (1999) Physiological pathways regulating the activity of magnocellular neurosecretory cells. *Progress in Neurobiology* 57: 625–55

Lieverse, R.J., Jansen, J.B.M.J., Masclee, A.A.M. and Lamers, C.B.H.W. (1995) Satiety effects of a physiological dose of cholecystokinin in humans. *Gut*: 36: 176–9

Lind, T. (1983) Fluid balance during labour: a review. *Journal of the Royal Society of Medicine* 76: 870–5

Linden, A., Eriksson, M., Carlquist, M. and Uvnas–Moberg, K. (1987) Plasma levels of gastrin, somatostatin, and chole-cystokinin immunoreactivity during pregnancy and lactation in dogs. *Gastroenterology* 92: 578–84

Lindstrom,T., Redbo, I. and Uvnas–Moberg, K. (2001) Plasma oxytocin and cortisol concentrations in dairy cows in relation to feeding duration and rumen fill. *Physiology and Behaviour* 72: 73–81

Lokrantz, C.M., Uvnas–Moberg, K. and Kaplan, J.M. (1997) Effects of central oxytocin administration on intraoral intake of glucose in deprived and non–deprived rats. *Physiology and Behaviour* 62: 347–52

Lopez–Luna, P., Olea, J. and Herrera, E. (1994) Effect of star-vation on lipoprotein lipase activity in different tissues during gestation in the rat. *Biochemica et Biophysica Acta* 1215: 275–9

Lyonnet, S., Coupe, C., Girard, J., Kahn, A. and Munnich, A. (1988) In vivo regulation of glycolytic and gluconeogenic enzyme gene expression in newborn rat liver. *Journal of Clinical Investigation* 81: 1682–9

Macho, L., Fickova, M. and Zorad, S. (1995) The effect of early weaning on insulin receptors in rat liver. *Endocrine Regulations* 29: 157–62

Magiakon, M-A., Mastorakos, G., Rabin, D., Margioris, A.N., Dubbert, B., Calogero, A.E., Tsigos, C., Munson, P.J. and Chrousos, G.P. (1996) The maternal hypothalamic–pitu-itary–adrenal axis in the third trimester of human pregnancy. *Clinical Endocrinology* 44: 419–28

Marcus, C., Ehren, H., Bolme, P. and Arner, P. (1988) Regulation of lipolysis during the neonatal period. *Journal of Clinical Investigation* 82: 1793–7

Martin, A.T., Benito, C.M. and Medina, J.M. (1981) Regulation of glycogenolysis in the liver of the newborn rat in vivo, inhibitory effect of glucose. *Biochemistry Biophysics Acta* 672: 262–7

Martin-Hidalgo, A., Holm, C., Belfrage, P., Schotz, M.C. and Herrera, E. (1994) Lipoprotein lipase and hormone-sensitive lipase activity and mRNA in rat adipose tissue during pregnancy. *American Journal of Physiology* 266 (29): E930–935

Martinez, V. and Tache, Y. (2001) Role of CRF receptor 1 in central CRF-induced stimulation of colonic propulsion in rats. *Brain Research* 893: 29–35

McCann, M.J. and Rogers, R.C. (1990) Oxytocin excites gastric-related neurones in rat dorsal vagal complex. *Journal of Physiology* 428: 95–108

McGarry, E.E. and Beck, J.C. (1962) Some metabolic effects of ovine prolactin in man. *Lancet* ii: 915

McLean, M. and Smith, R. (1999) Corticotrophin-releasing hormone in human pregnancy and parturition. *Trends in Endocrinology and Metabolism* 10 (5): 174–8

McLean, M., Bisit, A., Davies, J., Woods, R., Lowry, P. and Smith, R. (1995) A placental clock controlling the length of human pregnancy. *Nature Medicine* 1: 460–3

Menard, D., Corriveau, L. and Becaulieu, J-F. (1999) Insulin modulates cellular proliferation in developing human jejunum and colon. *Biology of the Neonate* 75: 143–51

Mendiola, J., Grylack, L.J. and Scanlon, J.W. (1982) Effects of intrapartum maternal glucose infusion on the normal fetus and newborn. *Anaesthesia Analgesia* 61 (1): 32–5

Miller, M., Wishart, H.Y. and Nimmo, W.S. (1983) Gastric content at induction of anaesthesia. *British Journal of Anaesthesia* 55: 1185–93

Mills, J.L., Jovanovic, L., Knopp, R., Aarons, J., Conley, M.,

Park, E. *et al.* (1998) Physiological reduction in fasting plasma glucose concentration in the first trimester of normal pregnancy: the diabetes in early pregnancy study. *Metabolism* 47 (9): 1140–4

Mirlesse, V., Frankenne, F., Alsat, E., Poncelet, M., Hennen, G. and Evain-Brion, D. (1993) Placenta growth hormone levels in normal pregnancy and in pregnancies with intrauterine growth retardation. *Pediatric Research* 34 (4): 439–42

Moore, K.L. and Persaud, T.V.N. (1993) *The Developing Human*. Philadelphia: WB Saunders, p. 98

Morien, A., Cassone, V.M. and Wellman, P.J. (1999) Diurnal changes in paraventricular hypothalamic α_1 and α_2-adrenoreceptors and food intake in rats. *Pharmacology Biochemistry and Behaviour* 63 (1): 33–8

Muchmore, D.B., Little, S.A. and deHaen, C. (1981) A dual mechanism of action of oxytocin in rat epididymal fat cells. *Journal of Biological Chemistry* 256 (1): 365–72

Mukherjee, S.P. and Mukherjee, C. (1982) Stimulation of pyruvate dehydrogenase activity in adipocytes by oxytocin: evidence for mediation of the insulin-like effect by endogenous hydrogen peroxide independent of glucose transport. *Archives of Biochemistry and Biophysics* 214 (1): 211–22

M'Zali, H., Guichard, C. and Plas, C. (1997) Time-dependent effects of insulin on lipid snthesis. I: Cultured fetal rat hepatocytes: a comparison between lipogenesis and glycogenesis. *Metabolism* 46 (4): 345–54

Nguyen, T., Diveky, L., Fedirko, B., Pak, S.C. and Parsons, M. (1997) Daily changes in plasma and amniotic fluid prolactin during the last third of pregnancy in the baboon. *Biology of Reproduction* 56: 597–601

Nakazato, M., Murakami, N., Date, Y., Kojima, M., Matsuo, H., Kangawa, K. *et al.* (2001) A role for ghrelin in the central regulation of feeding. *Nature* 409: 194–7

Neufeld, N.D., Scott, M. and Kaplan, S.A. (1980) Ontogeny of the mammalian insulin receptor. Studies of human and rat fetal liver plasma membranes. *Developmental Biology* 78: 151–8

Neumann, I.D., Johnstone, H.A., Hatzinger, M., Liebsch, G., Shipston, M., Russell, J.A., Landgraf, R. and Douglas, A.J. (1998) Attenuated neuroendocrine responses to emotional and physical stressors in pregnant rats involve adrenohypophysial changes. *Journal of Physiology* 508 (1): 289–300

Noel, M. and Woodside, B. (1993) Effect of systemic and central prolactin injections on food intake, weight gain and estrous cyclicity in female rats. *Physiological Behaviour* 54: 151–4

Nolan, C.J. and Proietto, J. (1994) The feto–placental glucose steal phenomenon is a major cause of maternal metabolic adaptation during late pregnancy in the rat. *Diabetologia* 37: 976–84

Nolten, W.E. and Rueck, P.A. (1981) Elevated free cortisol index in pregnancy: possible regulatory mechanisms. *American Journal of Obstetrics and Gynecology* 139 (4): 492–8

Odent, M. (1992) *The Nature of Birth and Breastfeeding*. Westport, CT: Bergin and Garvey, pp. 61–2

Odent, M. (1994) Labouring women are not marathon runners. *Midwifery Today* 31: 23–51

Ohana, E., Masor, M., Chaim, W., Levy, J., Sharoni, Y., Leiberman, J.R. and Glezerman, M. (1996) Maternal plasma and amniotic fluid cortisol and progesterone concentrations between women with and without term labour. *Journal of Reproductive Medicine* 41: 80–6

Olson, B.R., Drutarosky, M.D., Chow, M-S., Hruby, V.J., Stricker, E.M. and Verbalis, J.G. (1991a) Oxytocin and oxytocin agonist administered centrally decrease food intake in rats. *Peptides* 12: 113–18

Olson, B.R., Drutarosky, M.D., Stricker, E.M. and Verbalis,

J.G. (1991b) Brain oxytocin receptor antagonist blunts the effects of anorexigenic treatments in rats: evidence for central oxytocin inhibition of food intake. *Endocrinology* 129 (2): 785–91

Olson, B.R., Drutarosky, M.D., Stricker, E.M. and Verbalis, J.G. (1991c) Brain oxytocin receptors mediate corticotrophin-releasing hormone-induced anorexia. *American Journal of Physiology* 260 (29): R448–R52

Page, E.W., Villee, C.A. and Villee, D.B. (1981) *Human Reproduction: Essentials of Reproductive and Perinatal Medicine.* Philadelphia: WB Saunders, pp. 275–6

Pang, K.V., Newman, A.P., Udall, J.N. and Walker, W.A. (1985) Development of gastrointestinal mucosal barrier. VII. In utero maturation of microvillus surface by cortisone. *American Journal of Physiology* 249 (12): G85–G91

Parker, R.B. (1954) Risk from the aspiration of vomit during obstetric anaesthesia. *British Medical Journal* ii: 65–9

Patel, N., Alsat, E., Igout, A., Baron, F., Hennen, G., Porquet, D. and Evans-Brion, D. (1995) Glucose inhibits human placental GH secretion, *in vitro. Journal of Clinical Endocrinology and Metabolism* 80 (5): 1743–6

Paterson, P.J., Sheath, P., Taft, P. and Wood, C. (1967) Maternal and foetal ketone concentrations in plasma and urine. *Lancet* i: 862–5

Pearson Murphy, B.E. and Branchaud, C.L. (1994) The fetal adrenal. In Tulchinsky, D. and Little, A.B. (eds), *Maternal–Fetal Endocrinology.* Philadelphia: WB Saunders, pp. 275–95

Pegorier, J-P. (1998) Regulation of gene expression by fatty acids. *Current Opinion in Clinical Nutrition and Metabolic Care* 1: 329–34

Pegorier, J-P., Chatelain, F., Thumelin, S. and Girard, J. (1998) Role of long-chain fatty acids in postnatal induction of genes coding for liver mitochondrial β-oxidative enzymes. *Biochemistry Society Transactions* 26: 113–30

Pepe, G.J. and Albrecht, E.D. (1995) Actions of placental and fetal adrenal steroid hormones in primate pregnancy. *Endocrine Reviews* 16 (5): 608–48

Philipps, A.F. (1992) Carbohydrate metabolism of the fetus. In Polin, R.A. and Fox, W.W. (eds), *Fetal and Neonatal Physiology*. Philadelphia: WB Saunders, pp. 373–84

Phillips, I.D., Anthony, R.V., Simonetta, G., Owens, J.A., Robinson, J.S. and McMillen, I.C. (2001) Restriction of fetal growth has a differential impact on fetal prolactin and pro-lactin receptor mRNA expression. *Journal of Neuroendo-crinology* 13: 175–81

Phillips, I.D., Houghton, D.C. and McMillen, I.C. (1999) The regulation of prolactin receptor messenger ribonucleic acid levels in the sheep liver before birth: relative roles of the fetal hypothalamus, cortisol, and the external photoperiod. *Endocrinology* 140 (5): 1966–71

Philippe, J. and Missotten, M. (1990) Dexamethasone inhibits insulin biosynthesis by destabilizing insulin messenger ribonucleic acid in hamster insulinoma cells. *Endocrinology* 127 (4): 1640–5

Phillippe, M. (1983) Fetal catecholamines. *American Journal of Obstetrics and Gynecology* 146 (7): 840–55

Prip-Buus, C., Thumelin, S., Chatelain, F., Pegorier, J-P. and Girard, J. (1995) Hormonal and nutritional control of liver fatty acid oxidation and ketogenesis during development. *Biochemical Society Transactions* 23: 500–6

Quigley, M.E., Ishizuka, B., Ropert, J.F. and Yen, S.S.C. (1982) The food-entrained prolactin and cortisol release in late preg-nancy and prolactinoma patients. *Journal of Clinical Endocrinology and Metabolism* 54 (6): 1109–12

Ramirez, I., Llobera, M. and Herrera, E. (1983) Circulating triacylglycerols, lipoproteins, and tissue lipoprotein lipase activities in rat mothers and offspring during the perinatal period: effect of postmaturiy. *Metabolism* 32: 333–41

Ramos, P. and Herrera, E. (1995) Reversion of insulin resistance in the rat during late pregnancy by 72–h glucose infusion. *American Journal of Physiology* 269: E858

Ramos, P. and Herrera, E. (1996) Comparative responsiveness to prolonged hyperinsulinemia between adipose–tissue and mammary-gland lipoprotein lipase activities in pregnant rats. *Early Pregnancy: Biology and Medicine* 2: 29–35

Ramos, P., Martin-Hidalgo, A. and Herrera, E. (1999) Insulin-induced upregulation of lipoprotein lipase messenger ribonucleic acid and activity in mammary gland. *Endocrinology* 140 (3): 1089–93

Raygada, M., Cho, E. and Hilakivi-Clarke, L. (1998) High maternal intake of polyunsaturated fatty acids during pregnancy in mice alters offsprings' aggressive behaviour, immobility in the swim test, locomotor activity and brain protein kinase C activity. *Journal of Nutrition* 128: 2505–11

Rebuffe-Schrive, M., Enk, L., Crona, N., Lonnroth, P., Abrahamsson, L., Smith, U. and Bjorntorp, P. (1985) Fat cell metabolism in different regions in women. *Journal of Clinical Investigation* 75: 1973–6

Rigg, L.A. and Yen, S.S.C. (1977) Multiphasic prolactin secretion during parturition in human subjects. *American Journal of Obstetrics and Gynecology* 128 (2): 215–18

Rigg, L.A., Lein, A. and Yen, S.S.C. (1977) Pattern of increase in circulating prolactin levels during human gestation. *American Journal of Obstetrics and Gynecology* 129 (4): 454–6

Roberts, R.B. and Shirley, M.A. (1976) The obstetrician's role in reducing the risk of aspiration pneumonitis with particular reference to the use of oral antacids. *American Journal of Obstetrics and Gynecology* 124: 611–7

Roberts, R.B. and Shirley, M.A. (1980) Antacid therapy in obstetrics. *Anaesthesiology* 53: 83

Roberts, T.J., Caston-Balderrama, A., Nijland, M.J. and Ross, M.G. (2000) Central neuropeptide Y stimulates ingestive behaviour and increases urine output in the ovine fetus. *American Journal of Physiology*, 279: E494–E500

Rogers, R.C. and Herman, G.E. (1985) Dorsal medullary oxytocin, vasopressin, oxytocin antagonist, and TRH effects on gastric acid secretion and heart rate. *Peptides* 6: 1143–8

Rump, P., Otto, S.J. and Hornstra, G. (2001) Leptin and phospholipid-esterfied docosahexaenoic acid concentrations in plasma of women: observations during pregnancy and lactation. *European Journal of Clinical Nutrition* 55: 244–51

Sabata, V., Wolf, H. and Lausmann, S. (1968) The role of free fatty acids, glycerol, ketone bodies and glucose in the energy metabolism of mother and fetus during delivery. *Biology of the Neonate* 13: 7–17

Sangild, P.T. (1999) Biology of the pancreas before birth. In Pierzynowski and Zabielski (eds), *Biology of the Pancreas in Growing Animals*. Amsterdam: Elsvier Science, pp. 1–13

Sangild, P.T., Hilsted, L., Nexo, E., Fowden, A.L. and Silver, M. (1995) Vaginal birth *versus* elective caesarean section: effects on gastric function in the neonate. *Experimental Physiology* 80: 147–57

Sauve, D. and Woodside, B. (1996) The effect of central administration of prolactin on food intake in virgin female rats is dose-dependent, occurs in the absence of ovarian hormones and the latency to onset varies with feeding regime. *Brain Research* 729: 75–81

Schambaugh, G.E. (1985) Ketone body metabolism in the mother and fetus. *FASEB Journal* 44: 2347–51

Schams, D. and Espanier, R. (1991) Growth hormone, IGF-I and insulin in mammary gland secretion before and after parturition and possibility of their transfer into the calf. *Endocrine Regulations* 25: 139–43

Schneider, H. (1996) Ontogenic changes in the nutritive function of the placenta. *Placenta* 17: 15–26

Schulte, H.M., Weisner, D. and Allolio, B. (1990) The corticotrophin releasing hormone test in late pregnancy: lack of adrenocorticotrophin and cortisol response. *Clinical Endocrinology* 33: 99–106

Seccombe, D.W., Harding, P.G.R. and Possmayer, F. (1977) Fetal utilization of maternally derived ketone bodies for lipogenesis in the rat. *Biochemistry Biophysics Acta* 488: 402–16

Shamoon, H. and Felig, P. (1974) Effects of estrogen on glucose uptake by rat muscle. *Yale Journal of Biological Medicine* 47: 227–33

Shelly, H.J. (1961) Glycogen reserves and their changes at birth and in anoxia. *British Medical Bulletin* 17 (2): 137–43

Shelly, H.J. and Bassett, J.M. (1975) Control of carbohydrate metabolism in the fetus and newborn. *British Medical Bulletin* 31 (1): 37–43

Siaud, P., Puech, R., Assenmacher, I. and Alonso, G. (1991) Microinjection of oxytocin into the dorsal vagal complex decreases pancreatic insulin secretion. *Brain Research* 546: 190–4

Sidebottom, A.C., Brown, J. and Jacobs, D.R. Jr (2001) Pregnancy-related changes in body fat. *European Journal of Obstetrics and Gynaecology and Reproductive Biology* 94: 216–33

Simmons, M., Jones, M.D., Battaglia, F.C. and Meschia, G. (1978) Insulin effects on fetal glucose utilization. *Pediatric Research* 12: 90–2

Singhi, S.C. and Chookango, E. (1984) Maternal fluid overload during labour: transplacental hyponatraemia and risk of transient neonatal tachyapnoea in term infants. *Archives of Disease in Childhood* 59: 1155–8

Sivan, E., Homko, C.J., Chen, X., Reece, A.R. and Boden, G. (1999) Effect of insulin on fat metabolism during and after normal pregnancy. *Diabetes* 48: 834–8

Sivan, E., Whittaker, P.G., Sinha, D., Homko, C.J., Lin, M., Reece, E.A. and Boden, G. (1998) Leptin in human pregnancy: the relationship with gestational hormones. *American Journal of Obstetrics and Gynecology* 179 (5): 1128–32

Sjoholm, A., Sandsberg, E., Ostenson, C-G. and Efendic, S. (2000) Peptidergic regulation of maturation of the stimulus–secretion in fetal islet β-cells. *Pancreas* 20 (3): 282–9

Slen, S.B. (1969) Wool production and body growth in sheep. In: Cuthbertson, D. (ed.), *Nutrition of Animals of Agricultural Importance Part 2: Assessment of and Factors Affecting the Requirements of Farm Livestock.* Oxford: Pergamon Press, pp. 827–48

Slotkin, T.A. (1990) Development of the sympathoadrenal axis. In Muller, E.E., MacLeod, R.M. (eds), *Neuroendocrine Perspectives, 8.* New York: Springer–Verlag, pp. 69–96

Slotkin, T.A., Kudlacz, E.M., Hou, Q-C. and Seidler, F.J. (1990) Maturation of the sympathetic nervous system: role of neonatal physiological adaptations and in cellular development of perinatal tissues. In Cuezva, J.M., Pascual-Leon, A.M. and Patel, M.S. (eds), *Endocrine and Biochemical Development of the Fetus and Neonate.* New York: Plenum Press, pp. 67–75

Smith, I.D. and Bogod, D.G. (1995) Feeding in labour. *Contemporary Reviews in Obstetrics and Gynaecology* 7: 151–5

Soltani, K.H., Bruce, C. and Fraser, R.B. (1999) Observational study of maternal anthropometry and fetal insulin. *Archives of Diseases in Childhood* 81: F122–F124

Sorenson, R.L., Brelje, C.T., Hegre, O.D., Marshall, S., Anaya, P. and Sheridan, J.D. (1987) Prolactin (in vitro) decreases the glucose stimulation threshold, enhances insulin secretion, and increases dye coupling among islet β-cells. *Endocrinology* 121 (4): 1447–53

Sorenson, R.L., Brelje, C.T. and Roth, C. (1993) Effects of steroid and lactogenic hormones on islets of Langerhans: a new hypothesis for the role of pregnancy steroids in the adaptation of islets to pregnanccy. *Endocrinology* 133 (5): 2227–34

Sperling, M.A. (1994) Carbohydrate metabolism: insulin and glucagon. In Tulchinsky, D. and Little, A.B. (eds), *Maternal and Fetal Endocrinology*. Philadelphia: WB Saunders, pp. 379–400

Steingrimsdottir, T., Ronquist, G. and Ulmsten, U. (1993) Energy economy in the pregnant human uterus at term: studies on arteriovenous differences in metabolites of carbohydrate, fat and nucleotides. *European Journal of Obstetrics and Gynaecology and Reproductive Biology* 51: 209–15

Sterman, B.M., Gangull, S., Devaskar, S. and Sperling, M. (1983) Hypothyroidism and glucocorticoids modulate the development of hepatic insulin receptors. *Pediatric Research* 17: 111–16

Stock, S.M. and Bremme, K.A. (1998) Elevation of plasma leptin levels during pregnancy in normal and diabetic women. *Metabolism* 47 (7): 840–3

Stock, S., Fastbom, J., Bjorkstrand, E., Ungerstedt. U. and Uvnas-Moberg, K. (1990) Effects of oxytocin on in vivo release of insulin and glucagon studied by microdialysis in the rat pancreas and autoradiographic evidence for oxytocin binding sites within the islets of Langerhans. *Regulatory Peptides* 30: 1–13

Symonds, M.E., Phillips, I.D., Anthony, R.V., Owens, J.A. and McMillen, I.C. (1998) Prolactin receptor gene expression and foetal adipose tissue. *Journal of Neuroendocrinology* 10: 885–90

Tarnow-Mordi, W.O., Shaw, J.C.L., Liu, D., Gardner, D.A. and

Dlynn, F.V. (1981) Iatrogenic hyponatraemia of the newborn due to maternal fluid overload: a prospective study. *British Medical Journal* 283: 639–42

Tempel, D.L. and Leibowitz, S.F. (1994) Adrenal steroid receptors: interactions with brain neuropeptide systems in relation to nutrient intake and metabolism. *Journal of Neuroendocrinology* 6: 479–501

Tierson, F.D., Olsen, C.L. and Hook, E.B. (1986) Nausea and vomiting of pregnancy and association with pregnancy outcome. *American Journal of Obstetrics and Gynecology* 155 (5): 1017–22

Tourangeau, A., Carter, N., Tansil, N., Mclean, A. and Downer, V. (1999) Intravenous therapy for women in labour: implementation of a practice change. *Birth* 26 (1): 31–6

Tornehave, D. and Larsson, L-I. (1997) Presence of Bcl-X$_1$ during development of the human fetal and rat neonatal pancreas: correlation to programmed cell death. *Experimental Clinical Endocrinology Diabetes* 105: A27

Toufexis, D.J. and Walker, C.D. (1996) Noradrenergic facilitation of the adrenocorticotrophin response is absent during lactation in the rat. *Brain Research* 737: 71–7

Tschop, M., Smiley, D.L. and Heiman, M.L. (2000) Ghrelin induces adiposity in rodents. *Nature* 407: 908–13

Tu, J. and Tuch, B.E. (1997) Expression of glucokinase in glucose-unresponsive human fetal pancreatic islet-like cell clusters. *Journal of Clinical Endocrinology and Metabolism* 82 (3): 943–8

Turtle, J.R. and Kipnis, D.M. (1967) The lipolytic action of human placental lactogen in isolated fat cells. *Biochemistry Biophysics Acta* 144: 583–93

Uauy, R., Treen, M. and Hoffman, D.R. (1989) Essential fatty acid metabolism and requirements during development. *Seminary in Perinatology* 13 (2): 118–30

Uvnas-Moberg, K. (1989) The gastrointestinal tract in growth and reproduction. *Scientific American* July: 60–5

Uvnas-Moberg, K. (1994) Role of efferent and afferent vagal nerve activity during reproduction: integrating function of oxytocin on metabolism and behaviour. *Psychoneuroendocrinology* 19 (5–7): 687–95

Uvnas-Moberg, K. (1997) Physiological and endocrine effects of social contact. *Annals of the New York Academy of Science* 807: 146–63

Uvnas-Moberg, K., Alster, P. and Petersson, M. (1996) Dissociation of oxytocin effects on body weight in two variants of female Sprague–Dawley rats. *Integrative Physiological and Behavioral Science* 31 (1): 44–55

Uvnas-Moberg, K., Alster, P., Petersson, M., Sohlstrom, A. and Bjorkstrand, E. (1998) Postnatal oxytocin injections cause sustained weight gain and increased nociceptive thresholds in male and female rats. *Pediatric Research* 43 (3): 344–8

Uvnas-Moberg, K., Stock, S., Eriksson, M., Linden, A., Einarsson, S. *et al.* (1985) Plasma levels of oxytocin increase in response to suckling and feeding in dogs and sows. *Acta Physiologica Scandinavica* 124: 391–8

Vamvakopoulos, N.C. and Chrousos, G.P. (1993) Evidence of direct estrogen regulation of human corticotrophin-releasing hormone gene expression. *Journal of Clinical Investigation* 92: 1896–902

Van Aerde, J.E., Feldman, M. and Clandinin, M.T. (1998) Accretion of lipid in the fetus and newborn. In Polin, R.A. and Fox, W.W. (eds), *Fetal and Neonatal Physiology*. Philadelphia: WB Saunders, pp. 458–477

Van Assche, F.A., Hoet, J.J. and Jack, P.M.B. (1984) Endocrine pancreas of the pregnant mother, fetus, and newborn. In Beard, R.W. and Nathaniels, P.W. (eds), *Fetal Physiology and Medicine*. New York: Marcel Dekker, pp. 127–52

Van Cauwenberge, J.R., Hustin, J., Demey-Ponsart, E., Sulon, J., Reuter, A., Lambotte, R. and Franchimont, P. (1987) Changes in fetal and maternal blood levels of prolactin, cortisol, and cortisone during eutocic and dystocic childbirth. *Hormones and Research* 25: 125–31

Varma, M., Chai, J-K., Meguid, M.M., Laviano, A., Gleason, J.R., Yang, Z-J. *et al.* (1999) Effect of estradiol and progesterone on daily rhythm in food intake and feeding patterns in Fischer rats. *Physiology and Behaviour* 68: 99–107

Verbalis, J.G. (1999) The brain oxytocin receptors. *Frontiers in Neuroendocrinology* 20: 146–56

Verbalis, J.G., Blackburn, R.E., Olson, B.R. and Stricker, E.M. (1993) Central oxytocin inhibition of food and salt ingestion: a mechanism for intake regulation of solute homeostasis. *Regulatory Peptides* 45: 149–54

Verbalis, J.G., Blackburn, R.E., Hoffman, G.E. and Stricker, E.M. (1995) Establishing behavioural and physiological functions of central oxytocin: insights from studies of oxytocin and ingestive behaviours. In Ivell, R. and Russell, J. (eds), *Oxytocin*. New York: Plenum Press, pp. 209–25

Verbalis, J.G., McCann, M.J., McHale, C.M. and Stricker, E.M. (1986) Oxytocin secretion in response to cholecystokinin and food: differentiation of nausea from satiety. *Science* 232: 1417–19

Verbalis, J.G., Stricker, E.M., Robinson, A.G. and Hoffman, G.E. (1991) Cholecystokinin activates c-fos expression in the hypothalamic oxytocin and corticotrophin-releasing hormone neurones. *Journal of Neuroendocrinology* 3: 205–13

Vilhardt, H., Krarup, T., Holst, J.J. and Bie, P. (1986) The mechanism of the effect of oxytocin on plasma concentrations of glucose, insulin and glucagon in conscious dogs. *Journal of Endocrinology* 198: 283–98

Wauters, M., Considine, R.V. and Van Gaal, L.F. (2000)

Human leptin: from an adipocyte hormone to an endocrine mediator. *European Journal of Endocrinology* 143: 293–311

Wedenberg, K., Ronquist, G., Waldenstrom, A. and Ulmsten, U. (1990) Low energy charge in human uterine muscle. *Biochemistry Biophysics Acta* 1033: 31–4

Weinhaus, A.J., Bhagroo, N.V., Brelje, C.T. and Sorenson, R.L. (1998) Role of cAMP in upregulation of insulin secretion during adaptation of islets of Langerhans to pregnancy. *Diabetes* 47: 1426–35

Weinhaus, A.J., Bhagroo, N.V., Brelje, C.T. and Sorenson, R.L. (2000) Dexamethasone counteracts the effects of prolactin on islet function: implications for islet regulation in late pregnancy. *Endocrinology* 141 (4): 1384–93

Weinhaus, A.J., Stout, L.E. and Sorenson, R.L. (1996) Glucokinase, hexokinase, glucose transporter 2, and glucose metabolism in islets during pregnancy and prolactin-treated islets *in vitro*: mechanisms for long-term upregulation of islets. *Endocrinology* 127 (5): 1640–9

Widmaier, E.P. (1990) Changes in responsiveness of the hypothalamic–pituitary–adrenocortical axis to 2-deoxy-D-glucose in developing rats. *Endocrinology* 126 (6): 316–23

Widmaier, E.P. (1991) Endocrine control of glucose homeostasis in mammals: food for thought. *Molecular and Cellular Endocrinology* 75: C1–C6

Widmaier, E.P., Shah, P.R. and Lee, G. (1991) Interactions between oxytocin, glucagon and glucose in normal and streptozotocin-induced diabetic rats. *Regulatory Peptides* 34: 235–49

Wigger, A., Lorscher, P., Oehler, I., Keck, M.E., Naruo, T. and Neumann, I.D. (1999) Nonresponsiveness of the rat hypothalamic–pituitary–adrenocortical axis to parturition-related events: inhibitory action of endogenous opioids. *Endocrinology* 140 (6): 2843–9

Williams, C. and Coultard, T.M. (1978) Adipose tissue metabolism in pregnancy: the lipolytic effect of human placental lactogen. *British Journal of Obstetrics and Gynaecology* 85: 43–6

Windle, R.J., Judah, J.M. and Forsling, M.L. (1997) Effect of oxytocin receptor antagonist on the renal actions of oxytocin and vasopressin in the rat. *Journal of Endocrinology* 152: 257–64

Wirth, M.M., Olszewski, P.K., Yu, C., Levine, A.S. and Giraudo, S.Q. (2001) Paraventricular hypothalamic α-melanocyte-stimulating hormone and MTII reduce feeding without causing aversive effects *Peptides* 22: 129–34

Yen, S.S.C. (1986) Prolactin in human reproduction, In Yen, S.S.C. and Jaffe, R.B., (eds), *Reproductive Endocrinology*. Philadelphia, WB Saunders Company, 238–9.

Yen, S.S.C. (1989) Endocrinology of pregnancy. In Creasy and Resnik (eds), *Maternal–Fetal Medicine: Principles and Practice*. Philadelphia: WB Saunders, pp. 375–403

Yen, S.S.C. (1991) Endocrine metabolic adaptations in pregnancy. In Yen, S.S.C. *et al.* (eds), *Reproductive Endocrinology*. Philadelphia: WB Saunders, pp. 936–81

Zhu, Y., Goff, J.P., Reinhardt, T.A. and Horst, R.L. (1998) Pregnancy and lactation increase vitamin D-dependent intestinal membrane calcium adenosine triphosphatase and calcium binding protein messenger ribonucleic acid expression. *Endocrinology* 139 (8): 3520–4

Zumkeller, W. (2000) The role of gowth hormone and insulin-like growth factors for placental growth and development. *Placenta* 21: 451–67

CHAPTER FIVE

Eating and drinking in labour: the consumer's view

Louise Pengelley

- Place of birth matters in terms of eating and drinking in labour
- Does starving a woman affect the course of her labour?
- Consumers need adequate information to make choices
- Some Maternity Units are moving cautiously forward
- More research is required

The common practice of starving women is based primarily on a set of recommendations first published in 1946 by Mendelson. Much has changed in the labour wards of Europe and America since then, but this practice, a prophylaxis against aspiration pneumonitis or Mendelson's syndrome, has remained widespread. As a National Childbirth Trust antenatal teacher, I work for an organization committed to providing information and support to enable parents to make their own choices around the time of birth. In 1996 a colleague and I produced a briefing paper of current research to inform antenatal colleagues and prospective parents about the potential benefits and risks of women eating and drinking in labour (Pengelley and Gyte, 1996).

In the UK, women who book for home delivery are free to eat and drink at will, as are those women who choose to give birth in US birth centres (Rooks *et al.*, 1989). This contrasts with US hospitals where a postal questionnaire of the mid 1980s revealed that 47% of units had a NPO (Nil Prescribed Orally) policy, except for ice chips (McKay and Mahan, 1988). Recently a survey of 70 English maternity units found that 52.9% allowed food in established labour whilst 45.7% never permitted food (Berry, 1997). This contrasts with the results of a larger survey of UK maternity units which reported that in 64.7% of units food was never allowed in established labour (Michael *et al.*, 1991). The figure for permitting consumption of fluids other than water had risen, if slightly, from 44% in 1989 to 52% in 1994. Caution is necessary when comparing these two surveys because the more recent is so much smaller and confined to English units but an underlying trend towards more liberal eating and drinking policies is perhaps indicated. The author of the more recent study comments that questions about selection criteria of women for oral intake in labour illustrated a wide variety and many discrepancies between units. Midwives were shown to be 'poorly represented in policy decisions within units'. The author comments: 'increased midwifery involvement in policy making in the future may be instrumental in effecting greater flexibility of oral intake policies nation-wide ...' (Berry, 1997: 413–17).

In *Effective Care in Pregnancy and Childbirth*, Johnson *et al.* (1989: 827–32) state: 'the only justification for practices that restrict a woman's autonomy, her freedom of choice and her access to her baby, would be clear evidence that these restrictive practices do more good than harm ... and the onus of proof rests on those who advocate any intervention'. In other words, it is up to 'the intervener' to justify his/her intervention. In this case the intervention is preventing a woman from doing something that, given freedom of choice, she might choose to do during the course of her labour – which is to eat and drink. The crux of the matter is whether starving women does more good than harm. Does starving most women prevent death or illness in a few? Does starving affect the course of labour? Should all women be permitted to eat at will in labour or only those deemed to be at low risk of requiring a general anaesthetic, some of whom, of course, may later require anaesthesia for a caesarean section?

Mendelson (1946) recommended that labouring women (who in his time were encouraged to eat a hearty meal in early labour) should not eat in labour. This was to avoid, during general anaesthesia, often used for normal delivery in the 1940s, the twin risks of obstruction of the lungs by particles of food (suffocation) and of the syndrome named after him, the inhalation into the lungs of liquid acidic vomit. He also recommended that the contents of the woman's stomach should be rendered as alkaline as possible; that energy for labour should if necessary be given intravenously and that local anaesthesia should be used in preference to general anaesthesia.

The effect of labour on the movement of food and fluids through the stomach is still uncertain as no accurate method of measurement exists, but it appears from recent work using paracetamol absorption that active labour delays emptying of the stomach (O'Sullivan et al., 1985). Vomiting is common in normal labour, but, apart from being unpleasant, is of no clinical significance as long as the woman remains conscious. It is not established whether a woman is more likely to vomit if she has eaten but it is known that the longer she goes without food, the more acidic the contents of her stomach become (Roberts and Shirley, 1974). It is also known that narcotic analgesia, widely used in the UK and US labour wards, makes vomiting very likely whilst also slowing gastric motility to a virtual standstill (Nimmo et al., 1975; Nimmo et al., 1977; O'Sullivan et al., 1985). The risk to the woman is of her vomiting and then inhaling the contents of her stomach into her lungs as general anaesthesia is being induced or removed when the cough reflex is inhibited. In the words of two anaesthetists: 'it is this requirement for general anaesthesia that is the nidus of the problem of feeding in labour; no general anaesthetic – no risk of pneumonitis' (Smith and Bogod, 1997: 151–5).

Close attention to correct anaesthetic technique, and in particular the application of cricoid pressure, prior to the intubation of the lungs, along with good postoperative care, have been identified in the Confidential Enquiries into Maternal Deaths as the keys to preventing aspiration pneumonitis (Department of Health, 1991, 1994). The combination of a fall in the use of general anaesthesia in favour of regional anaesthesia (whilst overall anaesthetic use has risen with rising caesarean section rates) and attention to the high standards of anaesthetic technique advocated in the Confidential Enquiries has led to a sharp fall in deaths from aspiration pneumonitis from 37 between 1970 and 1972 (Department of Health, 1975), to 1 in 1991–3 (Department of Health, 1996) and none between 1994 and 1996 (Department of Health, 1998). Obstetric anaesthetists deserve credit for this impressive reduction in mortality from aspiration pneumonitis and thus from the tragedy that surrounds any maternal death.

The use of pharmacological methods, principally antacids and H_2-receptor antagonists, to reduce the volume and acidity of stomach contents, as recommended by Mendelson, is still widespread. All trials on these methods are small, ranging from $n = 18$ to $n = 117$. The reported outcomes relate to gastric volume and acidity, with no mention of maternal morbidity (Cochrane Library, 1998). Therefore, no relationship has been shown between their use and a reduction in mortality and morbidity from aspiration pneumonitis. The 1985–87 Confidential Enquiry (Department of Health, 1991) states 'the woman who died had received a commonly used antacid regimen and the failure of this technique to protect against the effects of pulmonary aspiration is disturbing'. The two women who died from aspiration pneumonitis in the next triennium, 1988–90, had also received full antacid prophylaxis (Department of Health, 1994). The 1991–93 report (Department of Health, 1996) describes aspiration of stomach contents as a 'potentially avoidable complication' of general anaesthesia for caesarean section. The use of antacid and H_2-receptor antagonist drug prophylaxis for all labouring women is discussed in the 1988–90 report (Department of Health, 1994) but only recommended for women requiring anaesthesia and those with pre-eclampsia. None of the reports states when any of the women described last ate or what they might have eaten, or discusses the potential benefits or risks of a woman feeding during labour. There exists no research to support starving a woman in labour, nor is there evidence that prophylactic antacids and/or H_2-receptor antagonists should be given to any woman except those at high risk of requiring anaesthesia. Yet the most recent survey of English maternity units showed that just under half did not allow food in labour (Berry, 1997), whilst an extensive survey of consultant anaesthetists, published in 1990, produced a figure of 75% using some form of prophylaxis against acid aspiration (H_2-receptor antagonist or antacid) for all women in normal labour (Tordoff and Sweeney, 1990).

Does starving a woman affect the course of her labour? Well-conducted research is badly needed to establish whether starving women influences such labour outcomes as length of labour, need for interventions (augmentation of labour, forceps, ventouse and caesarean section), the condition of the baby and the mother's perception of her experience. A recent, very small, randomized controlled trial showed no difference in the length of the first stage between a starved group and a group allowed a 'light standardized low fat diet' (Scrutton *et al.*, 1996). Plasma ketone levels and non-esterified fatty acid levels fell in the fed group whilst gastric volumes rose. Twice as many women in the fed group vomited, with a greater volume of vomit, but the small numbers in the study prevent any useful extrapolation to the general population.

Given real freedom to choose, do women want to be able to

eat in labour? A prospective descriptive study by Roberts and Ludka (1993) was undertaken to see whether, offered the choice, women would choose to eat and drink in labour. This was also a small study, undertaken in three hospitals in North-Eastern America and was not a randomized controlled trial, but its results are interesting. Of the 76 women who took part, all drank and 65 (85%) ate during labour. Fluid intake decreased as cervical dilatation increased but many continued to drink, with 20 drinking in the second stage of labour. Food was categorized into small, medium and large portions and half of the 65 who ate had medium to large portions, although only 2 ate in advanced first stage and 1 in second stage. Of the 'eaters' 80% did not vomit and 63% were not nauseated.

Another recent descriptive study from America was undertaken in a birth centre in Michigan where there are no restrictions on oral intake in labour (O'Reilly et al., 1993). As in the Roberts and Ludka study (1993), none of the women used narcotic analgesia. In this study a total of 106 women took part and all drank in labour. Oral intake was categorized into clear liquids, full liquids (such as soup and ice cream) and regular diet, i.e. solid food. Eighteen women took full liquids in early labour, 23 in active labour, 5 in transition and 2 in second stage. Fifty-five women ate solid food in early labour, 7 in active labour, 1 in transition and none in second stage. Twenty women out of the total sample vomited: 7 in early labour, 15 in active labour (but 5 of these had vomited before) and 6 during transition. Of those consuming full liquids, 1 vomited in early labour, 5 in active labour and 1 in transition. Of those eating solid food, 4 vomited in early labour, but none of the 7 who ate in active labour or the 1 who ate in transition vomited at all.

A pattern seems to emerge from these studies whereby almost all women want to drink and a majority want to eat. As labour progresses nearly all eat and drink less, with a few exceptions. The authors of these American studies expressed surprise at both the amount and type of food that significant numbers of women in their groups consumed. A relationship between type and quantity of oral intake and levels of emesis does not emerge from these studies.

In 1994 the National Birthday Trust performed a detailed study of planned home births throughout the UK along with a control group of women planning hospital deliveries (Chamberlain *et al.*, 1997). Women and their midwives filled in anonymous questionnaires about the delivery and their feelings about it. Of a total of 4191 women planning a home birth, who responded to the questions on oral intake, over 80% expressed a wish to drink during labour whilst of those planning a hospital delivery (3470), a similar 82.7% wished to be able to drink in labour. Of this 82.7%, 62.9% (1805) drank in early labour, 71.2% (2044) in mid labour and 44.4% (1275) in late labour. In the homebirth group 77.5% (2730) drank in early labour, 75.7% (2666) in mid labour and 50.5% (1778) in late labour. The hospital group were asked for reasons given to them if they were not allowed to drink. Of the 259 responding, 73 were told it was against hospital policy, 70 that they might need a general anaesthetic and 51 were not given a reason. There did not appear to be any choice at all for these women.

The wish to eat in labour, recorded before labour, was less strong than the wish to drink, perhaps reflecting the prevailing cultural view that women can't or don't eat in labour. So, only 33.8% (1416) of the planned homebirth group and 20.7% (718) of the planned hospital delivery group stated a wish to eat in labour. In fact, 89.7% (1270) of the 33.8% of the planned homebirth group ate in early labour, 35.4% (502) in mid labour and 5% (72) in late labour. In the planned hospital birth group 86.7% (623) of the 718 ate in early labour, 28.1%(202) in mid labour and 5.5% (40) in late labour. So, again a minority of women, a few in each group, chose to eat all the way through their labours.

Two hundred and sixty-two women from the planned hospital birth group responded to questions about why they were not allowed to eat; 102 were told that they might require a general anaesthetic, 51 were told it was not hospital policy and 42 were not given a reason. Between a third and half of those who did require a caesarean section had spinal anaesthesia, and among the total number delivered in hospital (i.e. including those transferred from home) only 2% of those who had eaten or drunk in labour had a general anaesthetic.

The City Hospital in Nottingham has, since 1994, implemented a policy of allowing women deemed to be at low risk of requiring a general anaesthetic to eat specified low fat foods in early labour. A multidisciplinary team comprising a research midwife, a consultant anaesthetist and a consultant obstetrician, but no consumer representative, wrote the policy and then with assistance from a dietician, compiled a list of ideal foods and drinks for labour.

Both the anaesthetist and the midwives involved have written about their initiative in Nottingham (Newton and Champion, 1997; Smith and Bogod, 1997). Their papers show differences in tone and emphasis that are perhaps indicative of the different perspectives on this issue to be found amongst most midwives and most anaesthetists. The Nottingham anaesthetists' paper reflects their anxiety and caution about the liberalizing of existing oral feeding policies (Smith and Bogod, 1997: 151–5). Whilst acknowledging that women may find starvation in labour stressful, that there is good evidence of the dangers of using intravenous glucose and that 'the risk of death due to aspiration is very small indeed', they go on to say 'the benefits of feeding are similarly nebulous and non specific. There is no strong, validated evidence that fasting in itself is a cause of morbidity'. And again, 'there is little evidence that withholding oral intake in labour is harmful, whereas death from aspiration pneumonitis, although rare, is a catastrophic event for the dead woman's family and dependants, as well as the staff involved in her care'.

They adopt a rather low key approach to the policy at the City Hospital in Nottingham: 'Based on current knowledge, in Nottingham the policy for oral intake in labour has been cautiously liberalized. Women are stratified into high and low risk groups. Low risk women comprise those in early labour and women whose labour is being induced. They are allowed specified solids and liquids ... but once labour is established, or if analgesia is required, access is restricted to the specified liquids only', and 'until more is known about the relationship between oral intake, gastric content and aspiration pneumonitis we should proceed cautiously'. The midwives' version (Newton and Champion, 1997: 418–22) is more optimistic in tone: 'as practitioners we wondered how we could promote the progress of a physiological labour without compromising the safety of the women in our care?'. The policy of allowing feeding in early labour was recently audited via a questionnaire (using open and closed questions) of 250 primiparous women. The objectives of the survey were to assess awareness of the policy amongst women and health professionals as well as identifying the appropriateness of the risk factors and usability of the policy. The audit showed that 75% of the women who ate during their labour (64.7% had been advised to eat when they went into labour by their community midwife), 22.4% (56) ate in hospital but 51.8% (128) ate at home and all but one ate when the cervix was less than 3 cm dilated. Use of analgesia, either pethidine (45 women) or epidural/entonox (167 women) was the principal reason for restriction of eating in hospital, or presumably being more than 3 cm dilated. However, the audit sought women's views and they said they appreciated having the choice and the reassurance of food and drink: 'it was nice to know I could, it's one of the yes things'. How much higher might the maternal satisfaction have been had they had the freedom to eat and drink at will throughout their labours? To a representative of the users of the maternity services, the policy in Nottingham is preferable to the enforced starvation endured by so many women for so many years in hospitals throughout the UK, but in allowing women to eat only in early labour, it represents but a small step forward. (This policy has recently been updated and is given as an Appendix in this book – see p. 141.)

Those who have written recently on this subject agree that research is badly needed into the effects of starving women in labour. It is crucial that any research does not exclude those women who use opioid analgesia, as this form of analgesia is so widely used by multiparous and primiparous low and high risk labouring women. Although Drs Smith and Bogod (1997) assert 'there is no strong validated evidence that fasting itself is a cause of morbidity', we do have a small but growing body of qualitative research to indicate that for many women being offered the freedom to eat and drink at will in labour makes a real difference to their overall labour experience. If, as the Nottingham midwives conclude, 'the use of analgesia appears to be the main reason why women cannot eat and drink in labour' (Newton and Champion, 1997), then perhaps the way forward, rather than continuing to withhold food from women, is to offer alternatives to opioid analgesia and epidurals that contain opioids.

The freedom to choose to eat throughout labour goes hand in hand with other recent developments aimed at improving the experience of normal labour; the freedom to move about, to have constant support from chosen companions, to remain upright and not necessarily use a bed, the use of water, massage, complementary therapies and TENS for pain relief. As with these choices, the decision to eat or not to eat in labour is partly about the woman taking control of her labour experience, having been given information about any proven benefits and risks. If she is to be advised against doing something she wants to do in her labour, such as to eat, this intervention can only be justified if she can be given research based evidence that by doing so she will be putting herself or her baby at risk.

Probably only a few women will choose to eat throughout their labours but it is already clear that many may appreciate the fact that the option exists. Whatever the actual events of the labour it is the woman herself who lives forever with the memories of the birth of her child. These memories, as any antenatal teacher or midwife knows from debriefing the labour experiences of her clients, range from being supremely empowering to, at worst, a sense of humiliation and failure, sometimes with severe negative psychological consequences. It is surely the duty of those who care for pregnant and labouring women to ensure that the woman and her partner can take as much control as possible of their birth experience. Having the freedom to be able to choose to eat if she wishes is an important aspect of giving control to labouring women. In the words of American midwives Roberts and Ludka (1993) 'it is worthwhile to note that food and fluids have many levels of meaning. One should be cautious in assuming that all oral intake is related to hunger and thirst. Food and drink not only provide nutrition but also have many positive social attributes. They can be a source of comfort for both the labouring woman and her support persons. The value of freedom of choice to choose and to assume some control over her environment should not be minimized.'

References

Berry, H. (1997) Feast or famine? Oral intake during labour: current evidence and practice. *British Journal of Midwifery* 5 (7): 413–17

Chamberlain, G., Wraight, A. and Crowley, P. (1997) *Report of a Confidential Enquiry of the National Birthday Trust of Home Deliveries in the Year, 1994*. London: Parthenon Press

Cochrane Library (1998) The Pregnancy and Childbirth Module. The Cochrane Library, Issue 3. Oxford: Update Software

Department of Health (1975) *Report on Confidential Enquiries into Maternal Deaths in England and Wales, 1970–72*, edited by H. Arthure *et al.* London: HMSO

Department of Health (1991) *Report on Confidential Enquiries into Maternal Deaths in the United Kingdom, 1985–87*. London: HMSO

Department of Health (1994) *Report on Confidential Enquiries into Maternal Deaths in the United Kingdom, 1988–90*. London: HMSO

Department of Health (1996) *Report on Confidential Enquiries into Maternal Deaths in the United Kingdom, 1991–93*, edited by B.M. Hibbard *et al.* London: HMSO

Department of Health (1998) *Report on Confidential Enquiries into Maternal Deaths in the United Kingdom, 1994–96*, edited by G. Lewis *et al.* London: HMSO

Johnson, C., Keirse, M.J.N.C., Enkin, M. and Chalmers, I. (1989) Nutrition and hydration in labour. In I. Chalmers, M. Enkin and M.J.N.C. Keirse (eds) *Effective Care in Pregnancy and Childbirth*. Oxford: Oxford University Press, pp. 827–32

McKay, S. and Mahan, C. (1988) Modifying the stomach contents of labouring women: why and how; success and risks. *Birth* 15: 213–21

Mendelson C.L. (1946) The aspiration of stomach contents into the lungs during obstetric anaesthesia. *American Journal of Obstetrics and Gynecology* 52: 191–205

Michael, S., Reilly, C.S. and Caunt, J.A. (1991) Policies for oral intake during labour. *Anaesthesia* 46: 1017–73

Newton, C. and Champion, P. (1997) Oral intake in labour: Nottingham's policy formulated and audited. *British Journal of Midwifery* 5 (7): 418–22

Nimmo, W.S. (1975) Narcotic analgesics and delayed gastric emptying in labour. *The Lancet* 1: 890–3

Nimmo, W.S., Wilson, J. and Prescott, L.P. (1977) Further studies of gastric emptying during labour. *Anaesthesia* 32: 100–1

O'Reilly, S. and Hoyer, P.J.P. (1993) Low risk mothers: oral intake and emesis in labour. *Journal of Nursing Midwifery* 38 (4): 228–35

O'Sullivan, G. and Bullingham, R.E. (1985) Non-invasive measurement of gastric emptying in obstetric patients. *Anaesthesia and Analgesia* 66: 125–8

Pengelley, L. and Gyte, G. (1996) Eating and drinking in labour. *New Generation Digest* March: 4–13

Roberts, C.C. and Ludka, L.M. (1993) Eating and drinking in labor. *Proceedings of the International Confederation of Midwives 23rd International Congress, 1993.* Vancouver: ICM 3: 1559–72

Roberts, R.B. and Shirley, M.A. (1974) Reducing the risk of acid aspiration during caesarean section. *Anaesthesia and Analgesia* 65: 248–50

Rooks, J.P., Weatherby, N.L., Ernst, E.K.M., Stapleton, S., Rosen, D. and Rosenfeld, A. (1989) Outcomes of care in birth centre. *New England Journal of Medicine* 321 (26): 1804–11

Scrutton, M., Lowry, C. and O'Sullivan, G. (1996) Eating in labour: an assessment of the risks and benefits. *International Journal of Obstetric Anaesthesia* pp. 214–15

Smith, I.D. and Bogod, D.G. (1997) Feeding in labour. *Contemporary Review of Obstetrics and Gynaecology* 7: 151–5

Tordoff, S.G. and Sweeney, B.P. (1990) Acid-aspiration prophylaxis in 228 obstetric anaesthetic departments in the UK. *Anaesthesia* 45: 776–80

CHAPTER SIX

Putting the evidence into practice

Penny Champion and Carol McCormick

- Cognitive dissonance about an issue stimulates action
- There is a change leader who has the support of a group of relevant and interested individuals
- Action research is used
- Change management theory is used

Eating and drinking in labour can be viewed from a variety of perspectives as presented in the preceding chapters. It is a challenge to consolidate the information and present a useful conclusion. Each chapter presents its own conclusion and all differ in some way. Only using one perspective will not provide us with balanced knowledge on which to base a clinical decision. One of the difficulties faced by midwives in the current practice climate is the need to provide women with information to make an informed decision. Historically, the knowledge base has been dominated by medically based research which perhaps accounts for the policy of restricting oral intake in labour. With the increasing body of information and research by midwives and colleagues working in other disciplines, such as psychology, physiology, sociology and women's studies, practitioners should be able to present a more balanced view.

There are still some very basic questions to which we do not know the answers, such as the energy requirement of a labouring woman (Enkin *et al.*, 1995) and how a solid or even semi-solid meal progresses along the digestive tract of a labouring woman. We may never know the answers to these questions. We do have a developing body of knowledge about the physiology of normal pregnancy and labour as evidenced by Chapter 4 in this book. Although complex, it does give us an insight into how incredible the body is in managing processes like labour, and that we need to take great care when intervening in such a finely tuned activity.

We remain in a situation where there is no certainty and no definitive answer to the question: is it safe for labouring women to eat or drink?

Professional ideology

The interpretation of research findings, and the use of other information sources, is deeply influenced by an individual practitioner's professional ideology (Lewis, 1991). It is not as simple as midwives believing birth to be a normal process and doctors considering it is only normal in retrospect. Practitioners' feelings will vary depending on their knowledge base, their experience and their confidence in expressing their opinions. In addition, practitioners are expected to work with several different levels of policy, such as the labour ward policy and the policies of their professional body, for example the Midwives Rules and Code of Practice (UKCC, 1998). Combining knowledge, personal views and policy documents in order to present meaningful information to a labouring woman is a complex process and there are sometimes conflicts to be addressed. Most midwives will be familiar with a policy, written or unwritten, of restricting oral intake for labouring women. For some, this restriction will be acceptable and for others it will conflict with their knowledge and/or their views. One of the key elements to change is education, and midwives who are used to a policy of restricting oral intake will need adequate knowledge updating if they are to accept and use a policy that liberalizes oral intake. This applies equally to medical practitioners. In a climate where research is constantly revealing new information we all need to accept that our practice is a dynamic, changing arena.

It is often said that medical practitioners have dominated and been responsible for the production of policy documents that affect the care of 'normal' labouring women (Robinson *et al.*, 1983). Before the importance of research based practice and multiprofessional teamwork in areas such as policy writing was really recognized, policy documents may have been based on the opinion of one consultant obstetrician or there may have been different policies on the same aspect of care for each consultant, highlighting the different ways of interpreting and combining professional opinion. Research based policy documents which are prepared by multiprofessional teams are an alternative and more objective way of guiding practice.

Individualized care

Policy documents are a means of guiding but also controlling practice. This is evident when the bodies such as Clinical Negligence Scheme for Trusts (CNST), who oversee risk management in maternity departments, ensure that certain protocols/policies are in place before they will allow Trusts to become members of the scheme (Dineen, 1997). Policies ensure that in the given situation a certain set of activities will take place and this should lead to favourable outcomes. There is no doubt that in an emergency situation a policy detailing research based activities that may improve the outcome is very helpful. However, in situations where there is no urgency such as oral intake in labour or 'slow progress' in labour, where there is not a generally accepted practice and where women can be involved in decision-making, policy documents as they are currently presented, impose a barrier.

How can a policy document which is written with *all* labouring women in mind actually facilitate the choices of individual women? There are two issues: the first is that the presentation of the information contained in a policy document which affects the care of labouring women needs to be more user-friendly and less directive, and secondly as practitioners in maternity care we need to think of policies as supportive and informative documents which help rather than hinder us.

Policy or guideline?

The information and opinions offered in the previous chapters of this book are an attempt to provide midwives and other professionals who participate in maternity care with knowledge to support their decision-making. It is unrealistic to expect any carer to have the time to read a book about each potential decision they may have to make. So, the information has to be presented in an available form, for use in the clinical environment. Typically this form has been the 'policy' document. In the case of eating and drinking in labour, these documents have either restricted or allowed oral intake.

In the case of eating and drinking in labour there is also the question of whether we need a guideline for practice at all. Jo Garcia and Sally Garforth (1991) in an extensive piece of work on midwifery policies and policy-making noted that 'there is no single answer to the question of whether policies are a good thing – for midwives, parents or other caregivers. What may be very important, however, is the active involvement of midwives in the process of policy-making and in the debates about the proper scope for policies in maternity care.' It seems that midwives have become increasingly involved in the formulation and writing of policy documents, but have they debated the issue of whether policy documents are a useful tool in achieving best midwifery practice? Have they had time and space to consider whether it is actually appropriate to have a policy about eating and drinking in labour?

One of the respondents in Garcia and Garforths's study said 'I have tended to get away from rigid "thou shalt" procedures and provided guidelines to good working practice. I feel that midwives must think for them selves and not always work by rote.' Some midwives and midwifery managers feel that having guidelines for *all* aspects of midwifery practice actually alters the practitioner's capacity for clinical judgement. If midwives always have documentation to guide their practice they have very little decision-making to do, and this has two negative effects on their practice. First it undermines their confidence in their ability to make a good clinical decision, and secondly, faced with a situation that is not usual, or perhaps in an unusual environment, midwives may be at a loss because they have come to rely on the hospital policies.

In many units midwifery practice is governed by a set of covert or unwritten policies and this has been the case with regard to eating and drinking in labour. Only one of the five maternity units in which one of the authors has worked had a written policy at the time, but the unwritten rule in all but one of them was that labouring women were not to be given anything but ice/water. The other unit actively encouraged eating and drinking, which was unusual at the time. If there is a covert policy which restricts eating and drinking in labour then having a policy document which liberalizes it is helpful in enabling midwives to practise physiological care. It also begins the process of changing practice.

Developing a guideline

How do we write a document that provides a practitioner with the information to facilitate informed choice, and which offers the practitioner the opportunity to exercise her or his clinical judgement. What we are saying is that the decision about eating and drinking in labour is for the woman and the practitioner caring for her to make, in the presence of the most recent and informative knowledge. It is important to note that a guideline about oral intake in labour should seek to provide information and to enable a choice to be offered. It would not be beneficial to develop a policy that encouraged women to eat and drink against their will; this would be no better than having one which disallowed them any oral intake. To use the words of Michel Odent (1994), 'we still have to accept that a woman's nutritional needs during labour are too complex to be managed by a birth attendant. Women must rely on what they feel ... to encourage a woman to eat noodles or add honey to her tea is no more appropriate than it is to impose restrictions.'

At Nottingham City Hospital the policy for starving women in labour in 1994 was an unwritten one. There was a certain degree of discontent among some midwives about this policy and this 'dissonance' led the research midwife to take up the challenge of changing it.

The change process and action research
The process that ensued was a form of action research. Action research is used extensively in social science settings and has many different definitions. Cohen and Manion (1994) offer us some insight into the usefulness of this method in changing practice: 'Action research is a small scale intervention in the functioning of the real world and a close examination of the effects of such intervention.' Other tangible features of action research are that:

- 'action research is situational, it is concerned with diagnosing a problem in a specific context and attempting to solve it in that context';
- 'it is usually collaborative, teams of practitioners work together on a project';
- 'it is participatory, team members themselves take part directly or indirectly in implementing the research';
- 'it is self-evaluative – modifications are continuously evaluated within the on going situation, the ultimate objective being to improve practice in some way or another' Cohen and Manion (1994).

Action research also demonstrates cyclical activity similar to the reflective cycle. There are a series of activities which the team move through in order to effect a change:

1 Planning
2 Fact finding
3 Execution
4 Reconnaissance.

This is based on the work of Lewin (1952), who also emphasized the value of involving participants in every phase of the action research process.

This theoretical background gives us the basic guidelines for a change process in clinical practice.

Planning

We have already noted the importance of a multidisciplinary team approach to the development of labour ward guidelines and in this case the midwife worked with a consultant anaesthetist and obstetrician as well as the labour suite working party. In other situations, the midwives have done the groundwork in terms of literature searching and compiling and then used various forums, attended by senior medical and midwifery staff, to begin the discussion process (personal communication, 2000/2001).

Fact finding

The process of compiling information to inform a guideline can take many forms. One of the key issues with making a drastic change in practice is that the practitioners who are going to use the policy are involved in the change and are educated during the process. For example, the labour ward working party may split the areas to be researched among individuals. This means that there are many practitioners around in the clinical area looking up information and sharing it with their colleagues and this begins the educative process. It also begins a process of change, raising people's interest levels, identifying those who are supportive of the change and using them to influence people who are not initially in favour.

In Nottingham, once the literature had been reviewed, the local conditions were assessed. The literature suggests two major risk groups for Mendelson's syndrome; women who have used pethidine and women who have general anaesthesia. The trend at Nottingham City Hospital was an increasing use of regional analgesia and anaesthesia and a decreasing use of opiate analgesia. These factors meant that, in light of the inconclusive evidence, liberalizing oral intake in labour was appropriate.

The advice of a dietician was then sought, to advise on food and drinks which would be appropriate for labouring women. These were foods which would be readily digestible, not increase acidity in the woman's stomach, would offer a good source of energy and were available on the labour ward. This list, shown in Tables 3.2 and 3.3 (pp. 40–1), necessitated skimmed milk, yoghurts and soups being ordered for the labour ward kitchen.

Bearing in mind that previous practice had been restricted by an unwritten policy that no labouring woman should eat and drink anything but sips of water, it was necessary to have some kind of written guidelines to illustrate the change in practice. These consisted of textual information and a flow chart.

The text gave a brief resumé of the literature, definitions of low and high risk factors, and an update about intravenous hydration and the antacid regime. Detailed information about the research background for the guideline was also available, but did not form part of the document. (See Appendix.)

The flow chart was a single page, which illustrated the course of action for women using different types of analgesia during their birth. When the policy was first produced in 1994, women who used epidural analgesia were restricted to drinks but this was challenged both by the audit which followed the introduction of this policy and by practitioners from other units who looked at the policy. This illustrates that guidelines are and should be dynamic and changing documents that are subject to regular review. This guideline was a compromise of opinion between several practitioners with differing perspectives. With additional evidence and some experience of how the policy worked in practice, those same practitioners had the confidence to liberalize the availability of food and drink even further. The current guideline is shown in Figure 6.1.

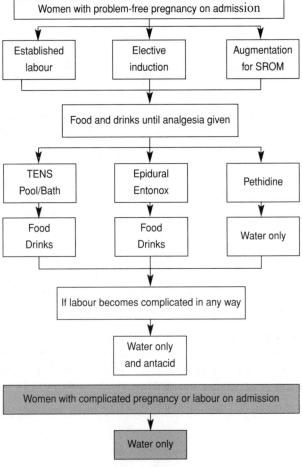

Figure 6.1 Current policy guideline at Nottingham City Hospital

Execution or implementation

Once the policy had been disseminated amongst the practitioners for discussion and their feedback received and addressed, the document was finalized and introduced into practice.

Time was allocated to raise the profile of the policy. Posters were put up in labour ward rooms and the guideline was made readily available both to practitioners in the hospital and community and to women.

Reconnaissance

An audit of the use of the policy was commenced, which collected both factual information about the birth experience and sought women's views, using a structured interview. The results of this audit are presented in detail in Newton and Champion (1997).

Following the audit project and a review of the policy in practice it was updated in 1999, so that women who were low risk but had had epidural analgesia could eat and drink.

This process enabled the production of a guideline for practice which was easily understood by both midwives and women. It alerted midwives to women who were at higher risk of aspiration syndrome according to the research that was available. Both women and midwives could clearly see the choices available to them. The options available to women were also communicated in a leaflet in the antenatal booking pack.

The policy currently in use in Nottingham City Hospital is an example of how the key issues of evidence based practice and multidisciplinary teamwork can work together to create a guideline that provides a stimulus for practitioners in thinking about their approach to each woman they are involved with.

Conclusion

Eating and drinking in labour is a symbolic issue in midwifery care, because it represents one way of 'normalizing' the care of women giving birth.

As practitioners in maternity care, our common goal is to achieve the best outcomes for all women and babies. We can only do this by working together, with women, recognizing each other's skills and acknowledging each other as equal partners in care.

Women-centredness is a crucial element in generating and implementing guidelines about an issue such as eating and drinking in labour. As practitioners we have a plethora of birth experiences which have very different meanings to us than they do to the women to whom they belong. Because of this difference, we create policies that have a huge impact upon women's experiences, but also have implications for women and their families which we do not necessarily consider.

The research by Mendelson (1946) which prompted the generation of restrictive policies and much of the subsequent work that supports these policies was undertaken using a quantitative positivistic approach which, it is generally accepted, produces reliable information. There is no doubt that work in this field has had some profoundly positive effects upon the safety of birth, in terms of reducing the incidence of Mendelson's syndrome.

However, this book has revealed a broader picture, using research and opinion that uses a more humanistic approach, favoured by the social sciences. By combining approaches we begin to be able to see the implications of the policies we create by only considering one perspective. Women's physiological and psychological experience of being starved in labour is slowly emerging.

Increasing knowledge of physiology supports the things we observe women doing in labour, such as eating well in early labour and not eating once active labour has begun. It makes us consider the implications of our actions on the transition of the fetus to extrauterine life. But, it must also humble us that our lack of understanding of such a complex process leads us to make some very inappropriate interventions.

The answer to the food and drink for birth question was never going to be a simple one. We must consider the feelings of the individual woman, all the evidence we have, including our clinical judgement, to facilitate the woman in making an informed decision. We can create and use guidelines such as those shown in this book but we must consider the implications and evidence for each woman rather than using them as a routine way of practising.

References

Cohen, L. and Manion, L. (1996) *Research Methods in Education*, 4th edn. London: Routledge, p. 186

Dineen, M. (1997) Clinical risk management and midwives. *Modern Midwife*, 7 (11): 9–13

Enkin, M., Keirse, M. and Chalmers, I. (1995) *Effective Care in Pregnancy and Childbirth*. Oxford: Oxford University Press

Garcia, J. and Garforth, S. (1991) Midwifery policies and policy making. In: S. Robinson and A.M. Thomson (eds), *Midwives Research and Childbirth*, vol. 2. London: Chapman and Hall.

Lewin, K. (1952) Group decisions and social change. In G.E. Swanson, T.M. Newcomb and T.M. Hartley (eds), *Readings in Social Psychology*. New York: Holt

Lewis, P. (1991) Food for thought – should women fast or feed in labour? *Modern Midwife*, 1 (1): 14–17

Mendelson, C.L. (1946) The aspiration of stomach contents into the lungs during obstetric anaesthesia. *American Journal of Obstetrics and Gynecology*, 52: 191–205

Newton, C. and Champion, P. (1997) Oral intake in labour: Nottingham's policy formulated and audited. *British Journal of Midwifery*, 5 (7): 418–22

Odent, M. (1994) Labouring women are not marathon runners. *Birth*, 31 (Autumn): 23–51

Robinson, S., Golden, J. and Bradley, S. (1983) A Study of the Roles and Responsibilities of the Midwife. NERU Report no. 1, Nursing Education Research Unit, King's College, London University.

United Kingdom Central Council (UKCC) (1998) *Midwives Rules and Code of Practice*. London: UKCC

Appendix:
Nottingham City Hospital Policy Guidelines for Feeding Women in Labour

NOTTINGHAM CITY HOSPITAL NHS TRUST

Policy Reference: Issue 3   Final Version

POLICY FOR FEEDING WOMEN IN LABOUR

Author Job Title:
Research Midwife
Consultant Obstetric Anaesthetist

First Issued on:
January 1994

Latest Reissue Date:
January 1996 (no change)
August 1999

Review Date:
August 2001

Document Derivation:
Policy for writing policies

Literature search

Consultant Process:
Labour Suite Working
    Party
Senior Midwives and
    Obstetricians

Ratified By:
O&G Directorate

Distribution:
Trust Board
O&G Clinical Director
Senior Midwifery
    Manager
All Maternity Wards &
    Departments

CHANGE RECORD

DATE	AUTHOR	DESCRIPTION	CHANGE RECORD
January 1994	Standard Setting Group	Diet and fluids for labouring women	January 1996 (no change)
August 1999	C McCormick D Bogod	Diet and fluids for labouring women	More liberal allowance of diet and fluids for low risk women

Status: Final Version
Policy Ref
Issue 1   Version 3

OBJECTIVES

To establish a mechanism and standard which takes account of legislation, guidelines and good practice.

THE NOTTINGHAM CITY HOSPITAL
FEEDING IN LABOUR PROGRAMME

Philosophy Labour is an energy-intensive process, but many maternity units deny calorific intake to women in labour (Michael et al. 1991), the justification being to minimise the risk of Mendelson's syndrome should general anaesthesia be required (Mendelson 1946). There is no research to establish the nutritional needs of pregnant and/or labouring women. Muscles only store enough glycogen for short bursts of energy production and therefore require regular input to maintain function (Katch and McArdle 1983). There is evidence, however, to suggest that a policy of starving women can turn a physiological event into a pathophysiological one (Ludka 1987).

The important aspects of gastric physiology to consider are emptying time and gastric pH. The policy aims to optimise both these aspects. The increased use of regional techniques for analgesia and anaesthesia has resulted in fewer operative deliveries using general anaesthesia and a decreased usage of opiate analgesia. This may well have contributed to the low incidence of Mendelson's syndrome.

With these ideas in mind a policy for oral intake for low risk labouring women has been compiled and is in use in the maternity unit of Nottingham City Hospital.

References

Katch, F.I. and McArdle, W.D. (1983) **Nutrition, Weight Control and Exercise**, 2nd Edition, Chapter Three, Lea and Febiger, Philadelphia.

Ludka, L. (1987) Fasting During Labour, paper presented at the **International Confederation of Midwives 21st Congress in The Hague,** August 1987.

Mendelson, C.L. (1946) Aspiration of stomach contents into lungs during obstetric anaesthesia, **American Journal of Obstetrics and Gynaecology,** 52, pp. 191–205.

Michael, S., Reilly, C.S. and Caunt, J.A. (1991), Policies per oral intake during labour: a survey of maternity units in England and Wales, **Anaesthesia,** 46, pp. 1011–1013.

Pengelley, L. (1998) Eating and drinking in labour (1), **The Practising Midwife,** July/August, Vol. 1 No. 7/8, pp. 34–37.

Scrutton, M.J., Metcalfe, G.A., Lowy, C., Seed, P.T. and O'Sullivan, G. (1999) Eating in labour: A RCT assessing the risks and benefits, **Anaesthesia,** 54, pp. 329–334.

Labour Suite

Guideline
Updated August 1999

Nottingham City Hospital NHS Trust

Maternity Unit

These guidelines are editorially independent of any
funding or bias.

GUIDELINES FOR ORAL INTAKE FOR WOMEN IN LABOUR

A comprehensive literature review including electronic data-
bases of information up to August 1999 reveals recent change
in obstetrics practice enables certain women with no problems in their pregnancy to have the option to eat and drink
in labour (Pengelly 1998). There is no research to establish the
nutritional needs of labouring women and there is a suggestion that starving women in labour may alter a normal physiological labour into a pathophysiological situation. Most of
the strategies in this area are aimed at the prevention of
gastric contents regurgitation and inhalation (Mendelson's
syndrome) which, at present, is very rare. Work by Scrutton
et al. (1999) suggests that feeding in labour reduces ketosis
but increases gastric volume. The two important aspects of
gastric physiology are: gastric emptying and gastric pH; and
current practice should be aimed at increasing, or at least not
to decrease both these functions, to protect the labouring
woman. The increased use of regional anaesthetic and anal-
gesic techniques has reduced opiate usage in labour and has
contributed to the decreased incidence of Mendelson's syndrome. The opiate usage was 20% of labouring women in
1997 at Nottingham City Hospital.

Gastric emptying inhibited by: pain, opiates, acidic foods (pH<3), high osmolality foodstuffs, fatty foods including milk, solid bulky foodstuffs, cold fluids (ice may be given in small amounts only)

Gastric emptying enhanced by: metoclopramide, cisapride

Gastric pH decreased by: antacids, ranitidine, cimetidine

LOW RISK WOMEN
Women with no potential obstetric problems and not using analgesia other than aromatherapy, massage, acupuncture, TENS, bath or birthing pool in labour. Or those having prostaglandin induction of labour not requiring analgesia and women with epidural analgesia for pain relief only in normal labour should be given the following advice about what they should eat or drink if they wish:

(1) SOLIDS: Low fat, low residue i.e. toast with butter and condiments (honey or jam), cornflakes, sugar and skimmed milk (<100 ml), plain digestive biscuits.

(II) LIQUIDS: Low fat yoghurt drinks, Tetrapack fruit juices (not: long life drinks especially apple, lemon, pineapple), tea with skimmed milk, soups (tomato, chicken, beef, squash drinks (not too concentrated), water, naturally carbonated mineral waters should be acceptable.

FOODS TO BE DISCOURAGED INCLUDE: Fizzy drinks (although CO_2 enhances gastric emptying these drinks tend to be hyperosmolar and excess gas may lead to abdominal distension and encourage reflux), full fat milk, Ribena[TM] and rosehip syrup, other drinks with high sugar concentrations, Lucozade Energy[TM] tablets etc. all solid foods, honey and jams alone, apple juice and other drinks with pH<3, alcohol.

© Nottingham City Hospital NHS Trust, Nottingham, UK. August 1999

ANTACIDS DO NOT NEED TO BE ROUTINELY ADMINIS-
TERED

LOW RISK WOMEN REQUIRING ANALGESIA
Women using nitrous oxide or an epidural (if the ONLY indi-
cation is patient request) should have only the fluids mentioned above.
(II) LIQUIDS in amounts up to 100 ml/hour.

ANTACIDS DO NOT NEED TO BE ROUTINELY ADMINIS-
TERED

HIGH RISK WOMEN
The following conditions necessitate restriction of oral intake
to small amounts of clear fluids only:
Opiate usage
Uterine scar
Multiple pregnancy
Breech presentation
Known IUGR
'Slow progress'
Trial of labour
Medical illnesses
Rhesus disease
Pregnancy induced hypertension
Antepartum haemorrhage
Suspicious or pathological CTG
Meconium stained liquor
Known anaesthetic problem

ANTACID REGIME
Ranitidine 150 mg, 6 hourly orally to the above mentioned
high risk women.

INTRAVENOUS HYDRATION AND NUTRITION
Intravenous fluids are not without complications for the

mother and baby. This is especially important in hyperosmolar solutions like 10% dextrose which should only be used to treat hypoglycaemia.

Index

Abdominal aorta, 71
Acid and gastric emptying, 33
Acid aspiration (Mendelson's
    syndrome), 2, 3, 12, 21, 29–30
  history, 13–18
  risk groups, 131
Action research, 129–30
Adipose tissue, 49, 54, 58
Adrenal medulla, 51, 71
Adrenocorticotrophic hormone
    (ACTH), 74–5
Alcohol, 13, 31, 34
Amino acids, 33, 34, 52, 61
γ-Aminobutyric acid (GABA), 48
Anaesthetists, 3, 15, 18, 20, 114, see
    also General anaesthesia
Anoroxigenic signals, 48
Antacids, 19–20, 47, 114–15
Anthropology, 11
Apoptosis, 60, 61, 65
Appetite, 48, 49, 52, 53, 70–1
Arachidonic acid, 56
Artificial rupture of membranes, 5
Aspiration pneumonitis, 14, 18, 114
Atrial natriuretic peptide, 50
Audit, 3, 133
Audit Commission, 5
Autonomy, 11

Birth centres, 112
Birth environment, 6–7, 112
Birth memories, 121
Biscuits, 41
Body fat, 35, 49
Brain:
  glucose requirement, 36, 71
  glycogen deposition, 58
  growth, 54
Bronchospasm, 17
Brown fat, 58

Caffeine, 34
Calcium, 52
Carbohydrate, 34, 35
Cardiac muscle, 58

Catecholamine, 72
Cell:
  death (apoptosis), 60, 61, 65
  maturation, 60
Central nervous system
    development, 56
Cereals, 41
Change process, 129–30
Changing Childbirth (DoH), 4, 23
Childbearing continuum, 1–2
Chloride, 52
Chocolate, 31
Chocolate wafer biscuits, 41
Choice, 115–16, 120
Cholecystokinin (CCK), 49, 50, 53
Chromaffin cells, 71
Cigarette smoking, 31
Clinical decisions, 128
Clinical guidelines, 5–6, see also
    Policy guidelines
Clinical Negligence Scheme for
    Trusts, 126
Cochrane Library, 23
Coffee, 31
Cola, 31
Comfort, 121
Confidential Enquiry into Maternal
    Deaths, 3, 12, 18–21, 114–15
Consumers, 3, 111–23
Control, 120–1
Corticosterone, 75
Corticotrophin-releasing hormone
    (CRH), 49, 73–5
Cortisol, 59, 60, 72, 75
CRH-binding protein, 74
Cricoid pressure, 3, 18–19, 114
Cricopharyngeal sphincter, 31
Culture of food, 11–13
Custom, 11

Dehydration, 36, 38
Diamorphine, 20, 32
Digestion, 52–3
Docosahexaenoic acid, 56
Dopamine, 49

Drinks:
  hypertonic, 34–5
  isotonic, 41
  for labour, 40, 41, 112, 131
  as treatment, 12–13
Duodenal villi, 52

Education, 125
Effective Care in Pregnancy and Childbirth, 23, 112
Eggs, 13
Emotional stress, 30, 75
β-Endorphin, 48
Energy requirements:
  homeostasis, 48
  labour, 37, 71
  pregnancy, term, 35
Epidural analgesia, 32, 131
Evidence-based practice, 2, 23

Fact finding, 130–1
Fasting, 22–3, 47, 55, 57, 115
  pH and, 34–5
  physiological consequences, 35–7
  stomach emptying, 31–4
Fatigue, 38
Fats, 31, 33, 34, *see also* Body fat
Fatty acid binding protein, 56
Fatty acids, 36, 54, 56, 57, 65
Fetus:
  hyperinsulinaemia, 39
  intravenous glucose effects, 39
  metabolism, 53–4, 55–6, 58–60
  pancreas, 60–3
  response to labour and birth, 71–2
Fish, 31
Flow charts, 131–2
Fluid requirement, 38–9
Food:
  cultural importance of, 11–13
  for labour, 41, 131
  preferences, 52
  as treatment, 12–13
Force feeding, 37
Fromage frais, 41
Fruit juices, 40

GABA, 48
Galanin, 48
Garlic, 31

Gastric emptying, 13, 15, 20, 21, 30, 32, 33, 113
Gastric glands, 34
Gastric juice, 34
Gastrin, 31, 34
Gastrointestinal function, 70–1
Gastrointestinal motility, 52
General anaesthesia, 3, 13, 15, 17, 19, 47, 113–14, 131
  postoperative care, 20–1, 114
Ghrelin, 48
Glucagon, 61–3
Glucocorticoids, 49, 65, 66, 73
Glucose, 52, 54, 61, 75
  brain requirements, 36, 71
  fetal and placental metabolism, 55–6
  homeostasis, 51–2
  intolerance, 65
  labour, metabolism in, 67–9
  powder, 17
  solutions, 34, 38–9
Glycogen, 35–6, 54
  fetal, 58
Glycogenesis, 58–60
Growth hormone (GH), 48, 52, 53, 59, 61, 63, 64
  GH-V, 64–5, 66, 67–9
  Guidelines, *see* Policy guidelines
Gunpowder, 13

H_2-receptor antagonists, 19, 114–15
Hair, 13
Heartburn, 31
Herbal concoctions, 13
High energy foods, 33
Home birth, 6–7, 112
Homeostasis, 48, 51–2
Hormonal regulation of ingestion and metabolism, 48–52, 63–6, 67–9, 73–6
Hospital birth, 6–7, 112
Hydrochloric acid, 34
Hyperinsulinaemia, 39
Hyperprolactinaemia, 64
Hypertonic drinks, 34–5
Hyponatraemia, 39
Hypothalamic–pituitary–adrenocortical (HPA) axis, 49, 73–6
Hypothalamus, 48, 49

Iatrogenic ketosis, 37
Ice, 17, 112, 128
Implementation, 133
Indigestion, 31
Individualized care, 126–7
Ingestion, neurohormonal
    regulation, 48–52
Insulin, 39, 51, 52, 53, 54, 57, 59, 61–3,
    66
Insulin resistance, 65
Intestines, 58
Intra-abdominal pressure, 31
Intravenous fluids, 38–9
    overload, 47
Intravenous glucose, 38–9
Iron, 52
Isotonic drinks, 41

Ketone bodies/ketosis, 36–7, 54
    placental, 57–8
Knowledge, 125, 126

Labour:
    energy requirements, 37
    fluid requirements, 38–9
    hastening, 12
    outcomes, 12, 115
Lactation, 52, 53, 57
Lactotrophes, 63
Leptin, 49, 53
Lipid metabolism, 54
    labour, 67–9
    placental, 56
Lipids, 52
Lipogenesis, 58–60
Lipoprotein lipase, 56, 57, 66
Liver, 36, 55, 56–7, 58, 64
    glycogen, 35
Lower oesophageal sphincter, 31
Lungs, 58

Malay women, 11
Mammary gland, 55, 56–7, 64, 66
Maternal morbidity, 12
Maternal mortality, 12, 21, 114
Meat, 31, 33
Medical practitioners, 126
Medicalization, 4
α-Melanocyte stimulating hormone,
    49
Memories, 121

Mendelson's syndrome (acid
    aspiration), 2, 3, 12, 21, 29–30
    history, 13–18
    risk groups, 131
Metabolism, 53–6
    feto-placental regulation, 59–60
    neonatal, 73–6
    neurohormonal regulation, 48–52,
        63–6, 67–9, 73–6
Metoclopramide, 33–4
Midwives Rules and Code of Practice
    (UKCC), 4, 125
Milk, 33, 34
    skimmed, 31
    synthesis, 57
Milking, 50
Mineral water, 40
Mist.Mag.Trisil B.P.C., 19
Multidisciplinary teams, 7, 126, 130
Muscle:
    glycogen, 35, 58
    protein, 36
    relaxants, 31
Myometrial contractions, 71, 74

Narcotic analgesia, 20, 21, 30, 32, 113
National Birthday Trust, 117
Nausea, 52
Neocortical activity, 71
Neonates:
    glugagon, 61–3
    metabolic adaptations, 73–6
Nerve cells, 36
Neuropeptide Y (NPY), 48, 49
Non-esterified fatty acids, 57
Noradrenaline, 48, 49
Normality, 4–5
Nottingham, City Hospital policy
    guidelines, 118–19, 129, 131, 132,
        133, 137–44
Nucleus tractus solitarus, 51

Oestrogen, 49, 53, 65
Oestrus cycle, 64
Onions, 31
Oroxigenic signals, 48
Osmolarity, 33
Outcomes, 12, 115
Oxytocin, 49–50, 51–2, 66–71, 73–6

Pain, 12

Pancreas:
  β-cells, 60, 61, 64, 65, 67
  fetal, 60–3
  maternal adaptations, 65–6
Parasympathetic tone, 53
Paraventricular nucleus, 50, 51
Pentazocine, 32
Peppermint, 31
Personal views, 125
Pethidine, 20, 32, 34, 131
pH, 29, 31, 34–5
Pituitary, 63, 67
Placenta:
  ketone transport, 57–8
  metabolism, 53–4, 55–6
  retained, 7
Placental lactogen (PL), 52–3, 59, 61, 63, 66
Planning, 130
Pneumonitis, 14, 18, 114
Policy guidelines, 4–8, 112, 125, 126, 127–8
  audit, 133
  developing, 128–32
  example, 132, 137–44
  implementation, 133
Postoperative care, 20–1, 114
Professional ideology, 125–6
Progesterone, 31, 53, 65, 66
Prolactin (PRL), 48, 52, 53, 57, 59, 61, 63–4, 66, 67–9
Protein, 31, 33, 34
Protocols, 4–8

Ranitidine, 19
Regurgitation, 31
Relaxation, 12
Research, 2–3, 8, 125, 126
Risk categorization, 119, 131
Royal Society of Medicine, 15

Scientific evidence, 2
Serotonin, 49
Skeletal muscle, 58
Skilled staff, 18
Smoking, 31
Sodium, 52
Sodium citrate, 19
Somatostatin, 53
Soup, 40, 41

Splanchnic nerves, 71
Squash drinks, 40
Staff skills, 18
Starving, 22–3, 47, 55, 57, 115
  pH and, 34–5
  physiological consequences, 35–7
  stomach emptying, 31–4
Stomach, 29–31
  emptying, 13, 15, 20, 21, 30, 32, 33, 113
Stomach contents:
  pH, 29, 31, 34–5
  volume, 29
Stress, 49, 71–2, 74–5
Suckling, 49–50, 51
Sympathetic system, 71
Syntometrine, 30

Tea, 13, 17, 40
Team working, 7, 126, 130
Temperature, 33
Textual information, 131
Thyrotrophin (TSH), 72
Time-of-day, 34
Toast, 41
Triacyglycerols (TG), 54, 56, 57, 66
Triglycerides, 66

Umbilical arterial blood pH, 39
Urine, 36, 38
Uterus:
  contractions, 12
  energy demands, 37
Utilitarianism, 4

Vagus, dorsal motor nucleus, 51
Vagus nerve, 34, 51
Vasopressin, 50
Verbal communication, 71
Vomiting, 16, 30, 52, 113, 115

Water, 17, 40, 52, 128
Winterton Report, 23
Withdrawal, 71
Women-centredness, 12, 134

Yoghurt, 41
Yoghurt drinks, 4